OMAD DIET

COOKBOOK

Effortlessly Transform Your Body Into a Fat-burning Machine

(Lose Weight and Improves Your Mental Clarity With Omad Diet)

Donald Marcus

Published by Alex Howard

© **Donald Marcus**

All Rights Reserved

Omad Diet Cookbook: Effortlessly Transform Your Body Into a Fat-burning Machine (Lose Weight and Improves Your Mental Clarity With Omad Diet)

ISBN 978-1-77485-009-1

Legal & Disclaimer

The information contained in this book is not designed to replace or take the place of any form of medicine or professional medical advice. The information in this book has been provided for educational and entertainment purposes only.

Table of contents

Part 1

Introduction

We've all been told that, in order to be healthy, we need to eat three meals a day. You should never, ever skip meals...or else. What if that accepted belief was wrong? What if you could stop counting calories and watching portions and still lose weight? Would you do it?

I realize that we're talking about breaking some of the dietary rules that we hold most dear.

Though it goes against conventional diet science, eating all your calories in one meal a day and still being healthy is a very real reality.

Intermittent fasting has exploded in popularity over the past three years. There are many incarnations of the principals. Essentially, intermittent fasting (or IF for short) manipulates you're eating windows by making meal times less frequent. This brings about a multitude of benefits, from easy weight loss, to better hormone sensitivity and increased brain function.

IF is not actually anything new – but has instead been something of a 'best kept secret'. From Hollywood diet gurus, to elite athletes, body builders and regular people like you have all switched to the one meal a day plan with amazing results. Why not join them? You'll be happy you did.

Who will benefit from this book?

This book is regarding a sustainable way to lose weight for overweight people. This method will work even if your weight doesn't let you work out in the gym. It will work even if you have lost all concern of losing weight ever. You can lose much weight and lose it fast.

If you feel that your weight has limited your life choices and it is degrading you as a person, then this book is for you.

If you feel that now is the time to lose the weight and live a healthy life, then this book is particularly for you.

If you feel that nothing has ever worked for you, then this book is just for you.

You will get to know the OMAD routine and the science behind it. This book will tell you the natural ways in which you can incorporate this routine into your life and get freedom from the life-limiting weight.

OMAD is the key to a healthy and joyful life. You can lose weight quickly and lose it harmlessly.

You will not be using any pills and won't require to pump iron in the gym for hours if you don't want to. This routine increases your metabolism and makes losing weight easy and fast.

No gain comes without some pain. You will have to put precise controls in place. Nevertheless, they wouldn't be tough, and with time they will grow spontaneous and simple. OMAD is a straightforward and time-tested method of intermittent fasting. It gives wonderful results in swift weight loss. You will not only lose a large amount of weight but steadily control it too.

If you possess a disordered lifestyle and you don't make time to work out, OMAD will work for you. If you have doubts about leaving some kinds of foods solely, OMAD will work for you. If you even have judgments about exercising pills for weight loss, OMAD will work for you.

This book will be your complete pattern to OMAD Intermittent Fasting. It will drive you through the science behind OMAD and the elements that make it so powerful.

It will also clear the conclusions about your strength to follow it. It will tell you the precise advantages of OMAD.

You will also get to know the exact method of utilizing the OMAD system in your life.

This is a complete guide to the One Meal a Day intermittent fasting, and I am sure it will change your attitude about losing weight conjointly.

One Meal a Day (OMAD) is the most sustainable and remarkable way for you to lose weight, even if all other measures have failed. However, you will have to put yourself together. In obese people, losing the weight is not the only challenge, maintaining it is an even bigger problem. People who go beneath the knife for weight loss cryosurgeries discover themselves standing in the identical place soon. One Meal a Day will not only help you in spending a lot of weight quickly, but it will further assist you in maintaining it effortlessly.

You need to read the book carefully and understand the effects of intermittent fasting on your body. The mechanics of food plays a critical role in our bodies and the One Meal a Day routine brings harmony to it. This book will help you in establishing a symbiotic relationship between your food and your body.

There are lots of books on this topic on the store, so thank you again for picking this one! Every effort was made to ensure it is full of as much helpful information as possible. Please enjoy!

Why we've Been Eating Three Meals a Day

"There is no biological reason for eating three meals a day."

Yale University Professor Paul Freedman

(Food: The History of Taste)

Freeman goes on to say that eating three meals and the scheduled time we eat them – breakfast in the morning, lunch in the afternoon, and dinner at night – are all cultural patterns.

The patterns of how we eat are no different than respecting someone's personal space or following a certain distance behind the car in front of you when driving. There's no science behind it – only long held patterns.

Naturally, marketing has also played its role. Take the breakfast cereal business – globally worth billions of dollars – and you'll see a small taster of the impact of marketing. Global brands like Kellogg's stand to make a veritable fortune by maintaining the breakfast status-quo. They spend millions of dollars pumping out adverts which highlight the 'heart healthy' full grains, the protein heavy nature of their foods and the calcium which positively impacts our bone health. They nag at parents to get them to support their child's health with a good wholesome breakfast. Yet in reality, it's all hogwash, manufactured marketing, with the aim of separating you from your hard earned money.

Then there's the simple yet understated impact of repetitive behavior.

Human beings love patterns because there's comfort in predictability. Before the electric light was invented, all meals were eaten during the day because cooking, serving, and cleaning up were difficult in the dark or by lantern or candle light. Once the electric light made its appearance, the later you ate became a status symbol. If you were well off, you could eat after dark.

In addition to the light versus no light rationale, through most of the 20th Century meals were planned around a worker's schedule. Farmers ate their biggest meal of the day ("dinner") at mid-day when they were done with chores. Factory workers ate at 5 pm when they could go home after a long day at work. As job roles and responsibilities shifted and families ate meals together less and less, the strict meal time structure also shifted. Since the invention of TV, meals began to revolve around what time your favorite TV show was on. After school activities gave rise to eating on the go and snacking instead of sitting down to eat a full meal. We no longer have time to eat three meals a day, so why be tied to that outdated pattern? Free yourself from convention and enjoy the health and weight benefits eating one meal a day gives you.

Health benefits of Intermittent Fasting

Intermittent fasting is an excellent dieting protocol that offers several health benefits. In this section, you will understand in regards to the different methods by which the diet plan will boost your overall health.

Weight loss

One of the primary benefits of intermittent fasting is weight loss. Intermittent fasting oscillates between periods of eating and fasting. While fasting, the amount of food you eat reduces naturally. Also it can help you shed weight and look at the same time. Apart from that, it also stops you from experiencing any type of mindless eating. Whenever you eat food, your body converts the food into glucose. The glucose which it needs is immediately converted into energy and the rest is stored within your body as fat cells. Not all the meals you take in become energy. So, each of the unused energy is stored as fat in your cells. When you start to skip meals, your body will reach into its internally stored energy. Once your system begins to burn fats to deliver energy, it automatically kick-starts the entire process of weight reduction. Also, most of the fats are normally kept in the abdominal region. If you want to reduce weight from the abdominal region, then this is the best diet for you personally.

Sleep

Obesity is rampant these days. In fact, it is a major health issue that humanity is experiencing. The primary reason for obesity in addition to a terrible lifestyle and food choices could be Insomnia. Intermittent fasting regulates your circadian rhythm and it encourages better sleep cycle. When the body is sufficiently rested, it is competent at burning fats effectively. A good sleep cycle has several physiological benefits like a rise in your power levels as well as an overall improvement in your mood.

Resistance to illnesses

Intermittent fasting aids the growth as well as the regeneration of cells. Did you know that the human body comes with an internal mechanism for repairing each of the damaged cells? Well, think of it as internal housekeeping that ensures that every cell in the body is performing optimally. When you follow the protocols of intermittent fasting, it raises the overall functioning of one's cells. So, it directly helps to increase the natural defense mechanism in the body and boosts the effectiveness against diseases as well as illnesses.

A healthy heart

As mentioned inside the previous chapter, intermittent fasting promotes fat loss. Burning up every unnecessary stored fat inside the body helps increase your cardiovascular health. The buildup of plaque inside the blood vessels is called atherosclerosis. Atherosclerosis occurs when fats start building up inside the veins. Also it could be the primary source of different cardiovascular diseases. Endothelium can be a thin lining present in the arteries as well as a dysfunction of this lining causes atherosclerosis.

Obesity is one of the main reasons to the build-up of plaque in the bloodstream; stress, and also inflammation, worsens this issue. Intermittent fasting provides help in cutting and removing the plaque deposits thereby helping to tackle obesity. So, this is the best diet in your case, in order to increase the health of the heart.

A healthy gut

Did you know your gut may be the home for a number of countless microorganisms? These microorganisms are helpful and so are essential for the best functioning from the gastrointestinal tract. These microorganisms are classified as microbiome. The gut microbiome is important for a healthy gut. A healthy digestive tract aids in better absorption of food and adds to the functioning of the stomach. So, a fairly easy diet change can assist you to boost your gut's health.

Tackles diabetes

Diabetes can be a terrible problem. In fact, it is right alongside with obesity as one in the leading health concerns currently. Diabetes can be another primary indicator to the risk inside increase of numerous cardiovascular diseases like heart attacks and strokes. When the level of glucose is alarmingly high in the bloodstream, and there isn't sufficient insulin to process the glucose, it causes diabetes. When your body starts developing capacity insulin, it can be quite difficult to regulate the sugar levels in the body.

Intermittent fasting decreases the problem of insulin sensitivity and effectively helps tackle and manage diabetes.

Reduces inflammation

Whenever one's body notices an internal problem, it powers up its natural defense mechanism - inflammation. Inflammation in moderate amounts is desirable and helpful. However, it doesn't mean that all forms of inflammation are great. Excess inflammation causes various health issues like arthritis, atherosclerosis and neurodegenerative disorders. Any inflammation with this form is recognized as chronic inflammation. Chronic inflammation is quite painful, and yes it can restrict one's body movements.

Promotes cell repair

When you start fasting, cellular structures in your system engage themselves in the entire process of waste removal. Waste removal refers to the entire process of deteriorating dysfunctional cells and proteins. This process is called autophagy which is quintessential for the repair of the body. Do you want to accumulate waste inside your home? Similarly, it can be important to ensure that the body doesn't start collecting any toxic wastes. Autophagy is the natural supply which reduces all unnecessary things from your body. Autophagy protects the neurons inside your brain from any cell degeneration. It not only protects the neurons, but also prevents them from excitotoxic stress. All these help the mind to replace the damaged cells with healthy new cells. When your body can do this naturally, it adds to the health of the brain. Autophagy also boosts the lifespan of cells and promotes longevity.

Improves memory

Intermittent fasting likewise helps boost your capacity to learn and retain things. Improving your memory is the best protective measures against neurodegenerative diseases. A diet that restricts the intake of calories helps increase your memory.

Reduces depression

Dealing with any mood disorder can be quite tricky. Medication isn't the only ways to take care of such disorders. A healthy diet that doesn't fill the body with unnecessary calories results in a total improvement in mood. Not just mood, it also improves your mental clarity and promotes alertness.

Don't always think of food

Regardless of whether to perform it consciously or otherwise, most of us usually keep contemplating just what the next meal is going to be. When you spend a great deal of the time considering what you would eat, you're essentially wasting your time and effort. For instance, let us assume that you are taking about four coffee breaks while at the office every break may last for about fifteen minutes. So, you might be wasting about one hour of your day being absolutely unproductive. When you are fasting, this time can be used to do other things. When you take away the dependence on food, it will give you the opportunity to be more productive. Not just that, in addition, it can help you concentrate on the job accessible rather than worrying about other distractions.

Better energy

People have a tendency to think that fasting for extended intervals will make them feel weak or perhaps sluggish. Well, that's most certainly not true with intermittent fasting. When you might be following protocols of this diet, you condition your body to start burning its internal reserves of fat to provide energy. Once your body starts to make this happen, then you will use a constant supply of your energy the whole day. So, even though you may not eat, the body keeps burning fats to supply energy. Usually, you observe a rapid dip in your efforts at around 4-5 inside the evening. This happens because the body utilizes the burnt glucose to deliver energy and the deficiency of it will make you hungry. However, when you begin following intermittent fasting, you do not notice any sudden dips in your energy levels and you may feel quite energetic each day.

Discipline

Self-discipline is important for fasting. Self-discipline improves your productivity. When you know the things that you must give attention to, you can do them continuously. Instead of whiling away your time and efforts on unnecessary activities, you are able to concentrate and improve your overall productivity. Not just that, it's going to even give you happiness. Self-discipline means that you'll be able to get the proper things done at the proper time. All this could make a happier individual. A person with self-discipline comes with more hours in a day than those without self-discipline. It doesn't imply you will definitely get extra hours per day. It merely implies that you have more time for it to do all the additional work if you don't procrastinate.

It enables you to decide what is right and precisely what is wrong. It enables you to distinguish between bad and good habits. Not just separate, nevertheless it even provides you the required willpower to do the proper thing. If you get sufficient rest and nutrition, your general health will improve. Self-Discipline can help you to stay healthy.

Different Methods of Fasting

16/8 method

The 16/8 technique is one of the easiest intermittent fasting protocols that exists. We are all effectively fasting while asleep, this technique is simply an extension of these fasting periods. Most of us have a tendency to skip our breakfast and often have our first meal after 12 noon. Well, on this method of fasting, you simply have to make certain that your eating window doesn't exceed 8 hours. In this method, it is necessary for somebody to fast for 16 hours in one day. The eating window is fixed for 8 hours. Two regular or three small meals can be squeezed into a day. This method is very easy to follow. It might be something as elementary as skipping breakfast; you aren't busy consuming anything after dinner. For instance, you can make sure the past meal that you've is at 8 in the evening. Make certain that you don't eat anything until 12 noon the next day. It provides you a fasting window of around 16 hours. It has been observed that it's better for women to fast for shorter time and don't let their fasting period exceed 14-15 hours. For those who feel hungry within the morning and are used to having lunch, this may be hard initially. However, if you're used to skipping breakfast, then it will be easy. You will surely have water, coffee and also other beverages that don't have numerous calories included while you are fasting. If you are going to choose intermittent fasting, then these will be the fasting protocol that you should consider.

5:2 Diet

If the concept of fasting daily doesn't interest you, then you can continue with the 5:2 dieting protocol. While following the dietary plan, the average person gets to eat regularly on five days in the week and restricts the calories to 500-600 calories, alternatively 48 hrs with the week. This diet is referred to as the Fast diet. On a two fasting days, it is recommended that women will need to have 500 calories and men can consume 600 calories. For instance, you get to eat regularly on all days except the two days whenever you need to fast. On such days, you are able to eat two meals consisting of 250-300 calories each according to your gender. This diet would work for all those who think they cannot fast for a whole day and who wish to have a little something to eat. 5:2 diet is often a very simple diet. You would have to decide the days in which you would like to fast alongside the days in which you don't. If you don't like thinking about abstaining from eating then this is well suited in your case. The days when you're fasting, you'll be able to either adhere to a strict diet or allow yourself to have around 500 calories.

Eat-stop-Eat

This type of intermittent fasting requires the consumer to fast for 24 hours, once or twice every week. You will fast every day and night consecutively on this diet program. From dinner of the first day until dinner of the next day, this will make it a day. For instance, you had your dinner at 7 p.m. on Monday, so you don't eat until 7 p.m. on Tuesday. This is going to be the twenty-four hours fasting window. You also can do this from breakfast of a given day until breakfast of the next morning. You will just need to fast every day and night; you'll be able to find the timings in accordance with your convenience. You cannot consume any solid food during the dietary plan. However, water, coffee and other beverages that don't have calories included may be consumed. If you're following this method because you would like to lose weight, then when this happens you will need to eat regularly within your feeding window. You must consume the type of food you're accustomed to eating, if you were not fasting. The only problem with this method is that there happens to be a 24-hour fasting window and yes it may be difficult for few people to check out. You don't necessarily need to start out using this type of fasting. You can gradually progress through the 16-hour fasting model. The first stretch in the diet won't be hard; it is only toward the end that the diet program becomes a little complicated to follow. This is where discipline and motivation come in handy.

If you continue to keep yourself busy, then you definitely won't have time to think about food or hunger. So, during the fasting days, make sure you keep yourself busy or engaged. Plan every day in order to enjoy all the activities that you're occupied with. You should have plenty of water. Not only will it keep your body thoroughly hydrated, but it will also leave you feeling satisfied. Make sure your week planned in this particular manner so that your fasting days won't clash with another social obligation. Intermittent fasting protocols may be convenient, and you must not compromise on your own dating life for that sake of the diet program.

Alternate day fasting

As the name suggests, this diet is all about fasting on every alternate day. There are different types of dietary plan. If you want, you'll be able to fast for 24-hours on every alternate day. There are some types that permit one to eat about 500 calories on every alternate day, while others require that you observe a strict fast on every alternate day. Most of the lab studies which were conducted to understand the benefits of intermittent fasting were made using different types of the dietary plan. A strict fast might sound rather severe and extreme. Depending upon your ease and comfort, you are able to adapt to the diet program for yourself personally. It is advisable that beginners don't immediately jump to the method. With this technique of fasting, expect you'll retire for the night hungry once or twice weekly. This diet doesn't show any form of sustainability within the long run.

Warrior diet

This form of fasting involves the use of small quantities of raw vegetables and fruit during the day after which consuming one particular hearty meal through the night. Mostly, you must simply fast throughout the day, and then you get to feast during the night. The feeding window reaches to only 4 hours. This variation with the intermittent fasting diets was one of the first to become popular. While after this method of fasting, the meal choices that you simply make should be quite similar to what you would have made had you been pursuing the Paleo diet. You will have to consume foods which are unprocessed. You can eat anything that our cavemen ancestors could have consumed. If something appears like it had been manufactured in a factory, you need to certainly avoid it.

The Paleo diet is often a high fat along with a low carb diet, just like the ketogenic diet. The protocols of the Paleo diet could be successful together with the dieting protocols of your intermittent fast. For instance, if you are following an alternate day type of fasting, that period of the days when you aren't fasting you must consume a Paleo diet. You just need to make certain whenever you are eating, the foodstuff that you happen to be consuming is Paleo-friendly. So, you cannot have any kind of junk foods, starchy foods or carbs. By combining those two diets, you can reap the benefits with the Paleo diet and intermittent fasting too.

Skipping meals spontaneously

Well, this is an obvious one and also this form of intermittent fasting doesn't have a very structured plan. You only have to skip meals spontaneously from time to time. Skip meals if you aren't hungry, or you are preoccupied with many works. If you aren't hungry, then don't eat. It is as elementary as that. Just skip lunch when you feel like it. Then determined by how hungry you might be until you are able to possess the next hearty meal. However, you will have to make sure the other meals that you are consuming are healthy. Skipping meals isn't identical to starvation. Don't make an effort to starve yourself, that's not what this method is about. By skipping meals whenever you aren't hungry, you're decreasing the unnecessary calories. Your body knows what it really needs and learns how to listen to it. Eat not until you are hungry.

One Meal a Day Diet

The interest in is increasing daily. One method of Intermittent Fasting (IF) that is steadily becoming well-accepted is the One Meal a Day diet also known as the OMAD diet. Abstaining from food helps modulate your system's performance and whenever you fast for prolonged periods, it provides a positive effect on the body and mind.

The OMAD protocol is designed in such a manner that the fasting ratio you need to adhere to is 23:1. It means that your system will be effectively fasting for 23 hours and also the eating window is bound to one hour. If you need to burn up fat, trigger fat loss, boost your mental clarity and lower some time that you simply devote to food; then eating one meal per day is really a brilliant idea.

The OMAD method oscillates between periods of eating and fasting. This method of fasting reduces the eating window a lot more than the other diets. After this dieting protocol, you have to make sure that you consume your day-to-day calories within one meal and you fast for the rest of the day. OMAD assists you to reap all of the benefits of intermittent fasting and yes it simplifies your schedule also. The ideal time for you to break your fast is between 4 and 7 p.m. When you do this, you allow your body sufficient time to digest the foods that you just ate when you sleep.

From the perspective of evolution, humans aren't designed to eat three meals per day. As mentioned earlier, our ancestor's bodies were functioning optimally regardless of food scarcity. Intermittent fasting protocols much like the OMAD tend to kick-start various cell functions in the body that are necessary to boost your all-around health. It is often rather intimidating to get started using this method of dieting. There are three simple tips that you can follow to generate the transition easier on yourself.

The initial thing that you need to accomplish is slowly cut back on the carbs that you take in. If you would like to optimize the outcomes of this diet and desire a minimal amount of crankiness, then you need to limit your carb intake. When consuming plenty of carbs, your system has a tendency to produce a stock of glycogen within the body. If some glucose is present in your body, then your body is not able to shift into ketosis. Ketosis is crucial to kick-start the whole process of burning fats. So, if you're trying to begin the diet plan, then this is a good idea to start out by slowly reducing your carb intake.

You must ease your body into getting used to this fasting protocol. It can be very tough to go from eating three meals per day to simply one meal each day. You have to ease the transition so it doesn't feel as if you're suffering. A simple way by which you can do that is slowly getting your system adapted to the idea of eating fewer meals. So, if you're used to eating three meals each day and often snack between the foods, then the first step would be to eliminate all the snacks. Then you are able to slowly increase the time between the foods and decrease the quantity of meals you take in. If you make this happen, it will be really simple to check out this diet.

Another simple way through which it is possible to make the diet program easier on your body is usually to consume some caffeine. A morning mug of coffee (lacking milk and sugar) could make you feel fuller longer and will keep your urge to eat away.

The Basics of the One Meal A Day Diet

There are seven basic steps or principals of the One Meal a Day Diet. If you follow these, you'll be in your way to a healthier and slimmer body.

1.Pick an objective weight range - Don't get involved with one specific goal weight number. Pick a range instead. Whether that suits you or not, your body is definitely in a very constant state of flux be it from water weight gain, age, gender, or some other factor. By selecting about five or ten-pound goal weight range, you're allowing yourself to get successful and letting go of your respective obsession using a specific number.

2. Weigh yourself once per week - It might be tempting to step on the scale every hour or every morning, but fight the temptation. Weigh yourself only once a week. The morning is right for weighings, especially before you consume liquids or food. Make certain to use exactly the same scale and try whilst everything is consistent as you are able to. Remember that weight changes will continually be linear because body fluctuations occur. The foods we eat, especially macronutrients, also can produce a huge difference. Sodium and carbs by way of example encourage your body's to hold more water weight, so if you take in foods that are rich in these compounds in the day you check your weight, you might register a higher bodyweight. You should look for chart out of the weight, and check out positive steps over weeks and months, not days and hours.

3.Pick a four hour time window to your one meal - Early evenings from 4-8 pm is generally the best time to eat your everyday calorie intake, but it is possible to pick any four hour window in the daytime. The important thing would be to never desist from this time around the window.

4. Remember the "four ONES" - These would be the nuts and bolts in the one meal per day diet. (1) Only ONE meal per day. No snacking on anything with calories afterward. Eat just as much as you desire. (2) Only ONE regular size dinner plate filled completely. Don't eat from packages or containers. Fill your plate

completely with foods - desserts and you will be able to work with 1,700 calories on the plate. (3) Only ONE caloric drink with all the meal. Anyone 12 to 16-ounce caloric drink will perform. Beer, soda, milk, juice. Save the non-caloric drinks for after your meal. (4) Finish your meal within ONE hour. Don't graze for four hours straight. Fill your plate together with your 1,700 calories and take care of within 60 minutes.

5. Drink non-caloric drinks after your meal - Coffee, tea, and plain water would be the top choices for the zero calorie beverages. You can also do diet soda and flavored water (NB we do not encourage you to consume way too many diet sodas. The medical issues surrounding these options are still not fully understood, however when it comes to dieting and cutting excess fat, a lot of people think they are doing help. Did you know how many models and bodybuilders use diet coke to kill food cravings and food cravings?). Vary the kind beverages you drink so your system doesn't raise your capacity anything.

6. Have some days to splurge yourself every week - Ignore the one plate/one drink rules. Don't stuff yourself, but it's okay should you choose. It's a splurge day! The calorie splurge can help kick your metabolism into higher gear making up for virtually any calories you could be under the rest from the week. Some of our clients want to make use of this splurge. You can eat multiple meals a day. To illustrate, I like to take lunch with my team members over the Friday. We

make a problem from the jaw horse and check out nice bars and restaurants. Done sparingly, this will really help what you eat and weight reduction goals and I still find it helps me to remain motivated for the next week.

7. Don't stray from any of the rules above - The first week will probably be the hardest. You might feel shaky and hungry but this will likely pass as one's body detoxes and adjusts to your new lifestyle. The benefits of breaking the meat addiction outweigh a symptom 'hiccups' whilst you adapt to it. If you're used to a really high volume of meals - several of my bodybuilding customers are used to eating six meals each day! - You then may desire to phase yourself straight into this way of eating. Start with reducing breakfast and some other meals before lunch. Then slowly work on pushing your lunch backward when you're not eating until 4 pm. Then as time passes you can develop merging lunch and dinner, at which you'll be in your one meal per day regime.

What to Expect When Starting OMAD

When beginning OMAD diets, the initial thing most people experience is hunger so you are not alone. This is probably a problem of body conditioning that you simply ought to battle the first few weeks. You may not really be hungry, but because you might have been eating repeatedly per day, your system may be trained to expect food every few hours.

While this can change from one person to another, a "fasting headache" is typical for your first few weeks. This is triggered by the mixture of low blood glucose levels, dehydration, and perchance lack of sleep. The trick is to keep yourself hydrated throughout your fast.

The brain is 75% water and is also very responsive to dehydration, and produced histamines to ration and conserve water when faced with a shortage. It is these histamines that cause headaches along with fatigues; these are an indication that we need to drink more water. Keep in mind that this discomfort can finish once your body gets used to your eating schedule as well as the deficiency of intermittent snacks during the day.

Keeping yourself busy with work or distracting yourself by immersing yourself in other pursuits can help you think less about food. Staying away through the kitchen or pantry will even help, as you do continually see and smell food to whet your appetite when it is not your meal time.

Once the mind has been disciplined to eat only meal a day, one's body will adjust eventually.

The Key to Going OMAD Successfully

Since successful weight reduction with all the OMAD diet requires that you restrict your intake of calories if you want to slim down and realize some form the benefits that are associated with the diet; having some insight on what the macronutrients are is therefore vital.

Here is definitely an overview of the macronutrients that the body needs in order to function better.

Protein: When working out, the muscles essentially stop working and your system requires protein for building muscles and recovering from the training. While it is commonly present in meat and dairy, protein may also be found in nuts and legumes. The rule of thumb for athletes and bodybuilders is to get 1 gram of protein for each pound of bodyweight. Each gram of protein comes to 4 calories.

Carbohydrates: Carbohydrates aka carbs will be the body's main source of energy, and if comprises fiber, starch, and sugar.

Simple carbohydrates are generally made available to the bloodstream faster and spark a spike in blood sugar levels. Sugar is often a simple carbohydrate.

Complex carbohydrates are more difficult to digest and are absorbed into the bloodstream slowly. They don't result in a spike in blood glucose. Fiber and starch are complex carbohydrates.

Each gram of carbohydrate matches 4 calories and the sources of calories are grain, bread, pasta, rice, potatoes, and sugar.

Fats: Fats will also be essential for optimal body health and yes it gives your body a store of energy. Fat can be necessary to maintain your skin and hair healthy, and also to absorb certain fat-soluble vitamins. There are three forms of fats: fats, unsaturated fats, and trans fat.

Saturated fats can lift up your LDL (bad cholesterol), and an excessive amount it may place you prone to serious health problems like heart attack and stroke. Foods which are high in saturated fats are dairy and animal products.

Unsaturated fats can reduce your LDL. They are found mainly in vegetable oil such as extra virgin, olive oil and canola oil.

Trans fats would be the result of vegetable oil hardening and will both increase your LDL (bad cholesterol) and lower your HDL (good cholesterol). Avoid these anywhere possible. Trans fats may be present in margarine, microwave popcorn, frozen pizza, plus some cake frosting.

Caloric maintenance: Caloric maintenance could be the number of calories that your system requires each day in order to become in the state where it doesn't lose or put on weight. Caloric gain has a tendency to consist of person to person with factors like age, gender, muscular mass, and lifestyle needing to be taken into consideration.

If you want to shed weight then this calorie consumption should be less than what your body expends every day. Each pound of bodyweight is roughly 3,500 calories. To find your recommended caloric intake, you'll be able to use a web-based calorie calculator.

How the OMAD Routine Works

Weight loss can be a complex process. As the saying goes, "Rome wasn't built in a day," and also the same goes for your accumulated weight and fat. The excess weight and fat have been piling up for a long time. Mostly, fat accumulation is as a result of the negligence of your lifestyle choices. Here, with the word 'mostly' is key, as it is not the only reason that can bring about weight gain.

Genetic problems, other medical issues leading to immobility and hormonal issues could also result in weight gain. However, this book is about putting on weight issues in individuals who have gained unwanted weight and abdominal fat due to poor lifestyle choices. Therefore, we'll stick to it.

Our body has a very sophisticated and detailed system of functioning. It is vital that you comprehend the way your body functions to comprehend the complexities that cause excess fat gain. The first concept to know is that one's body doesn't look at weight as a liability but a good point.

Like all other organisms within this blue planet, individuals were also developed to survive for long periods. The food is a prized commodity for all creatures, so it was for mankind. In the start and, until the previous centuries, getting food has not been so easy. Men were required to set up a fight against beasts to have every morsel of food. It was tough, where there was no certainty. There were seasons of feasts and famines. Our body has a system of accumulating energy as fat to survive the times of famines. This fat is employed in occasions when there is certainly no supply of food. This mechanism continues to be employed for all other beings. However, there has been a slight change for mankind within this regard. The seasons of famines have almost ceased to exist because of the abundance of food through modernization. This mechanism remains to be set up and functioning.

When you consume anything, your body processes that food into glucose. Your body then assesses the actual requirement for energy. The required energy passes to your bloodstream by means of blood glucose. All your organs and cells can access this as direct energy. Your pancreas gets to work and releases the hormone insulin which enables the cells to absorb this energy. However, in the event, the energy produced is greater than is required. The body stores that extra energy by means of glycogen. This is directly saved in the liver and muscles. The insulin present inside your blood will direct this transformation. However, when the present energy is really a lot above the amount which can be stored as glycogen, it is being stored as fat. Insulin sends signals to the fat stores and places the extra energy available as fat cells. This is the process of accumulation of visceral fat, body fat around your belly, thighs, hips, and each of the odd places.

Now, there is often a fundamental question here. When our own bodies have this efficient system, why doesn't it target this fat by itself? Why is burning this visceral fat so tricky? Here, you ought to return on the earlier point that our body's following a feast and famine system. The fat stores within the body aren't a liability, but a good thing for your body. Our body efforts to keep fat stored intact is being used inside the rainy days when food is scarce. However, those times rarely appear in contemporary society. In today's reality, that fat is often a liability for you. Your body will never try to burn these fat stored without treatment until it necessarily feels the need to accomplish so.

The truth is clear that one's body won't burn this excess fat until it can be forced to accomplish so. If you think that by dieting or exercising in the usual way you are able to force your body to lose this beloved fat, then you're mistaken. Your body will simply take these steps if it finds which the issue is.

Our body will burn the challenging visceral fat only once it can be in dire need of energy. This can't happen while you keep feeding it with more food at regular intervals. Therefore, intermittent fasting is the greatest way to cut this continuous supply of easily available energy to your body. It assists you to in forcing your body to begin burning the fat stored that will supply clean energy to your body. However, there can be a big misconception that intermittent fasting, for that matter; any fasting can make you weak.

Once again, think of our ancestors. They were hunter-gatherer nomads. There was no shortage of food on their behalf. With their primitive weapons and limited knowledge, the percentages of having food over a daily basis were low. However, their health needed more strength on the times after they didn't have food for long periods, to hunt more aggressively. Their minds required to think more clearly on the periods they didn't get food. If not, their odds of having any longer food would reduce drastically. Therefore, the misconception how the not enough food for a long time of fasting could make you weak or get rid of the clarity of thoughts is wrong. Once your ready supply of energy is cut-off, the body will switch to burning the fat for energy. It needs to get even stronger and much more robust on days past to survive in a hostile environment.

Intermittent fasting could be the way the body is actually meant to function by Mother Nature. Your work schedule and kind of job won't be a problem. Your energy needs may also be no factor when considering intermittent fasting as you get the required amount of your energy inside your eating windows. The OMAD routine of intermittent fasting will give you an eating window to ensure that you'll be able to receive the supply of their time needed. This will be sure that the body doesn't feel it's in the starvation situation. Nevertheless, it helps to keep your body in the fasted state for long enough so it feels the need to get started on burning the fat stores. Whether you might be performing a white-collar job which has a 9 to 5 shift or pumping iron within the gym for bodybuilding, intermittent fasting can work for those.

It is the best and most successful method to reduce weight and burn the tough belly fat. The OMAD routine gives the body a fasting window of 20+ hours. This fasting window helps with increasing the weight reduction and weight loss procedure.

The OMAD routine also offers many health advantages. It has incredible anti-aging benefits and improves your overall health biomarkers. This routine improves your insulin sensitivity and cures the chronic inflammation in the fat cells.

Following the OMAD Routine

We have discussed in more details the items OMAD routine are able to do to suit your needs. It can bring an alternative change in your life and make you appear and feel a lot better. You understand that you just feel far healthier and comfortable inside your skin. Although this all sounds good, remaining hungry with an extended period still seems somewhat intimidating.

If you are concerned with being hungry on an extended period, you then must hold your horses a little. Suddenly starting the OMAD routine is neither required nor suggested. Switching to long fasting hours at the same time isn't recommended. Your body has been running on quick, cheap energy supplied by carbohydrates. To burn fat and remain energetic, the body will have to get 'Keto-Adapted.' This process needs time to work and patience. If you attempt to rush this process of extended fasting, there are chances that your system will suffer control and may even start munching on parts of your muscles too. Your blood glucose also can get low, understanding that isn't healthy either. You must come up with a slow transition. You will have to train yourself to keep on without food, slowly and gradually. Once the body gets confident with one degree of fasting, only then you should move towards the next level.

3 Meals a Day without Snacking in-between

At first, you can start training one's body to keep on three meals a day. This means it is possible to have breakfast, lunch, and dinner at usual timings. However, you have to not consume whatever else inside the day. There should be no snacks or munching in the daytime besides those three meals. This isn't a fasting routine since the gap between the foods will likely be 4-5 hours. However, this is often a good and healthy start, as gives the body time to assimilate. You can follow this routine unless you don't feel hungry between meals. The OMAD routine is a discipline. Every discipline needs training and patience. It is often a procedure that needs to become followed with consistency. If you attempt to rush the process, then you definitely may lose control midway. Therefore, it can be vital that you simply first distance yourself through the extra snacking you might have been doing. This will perform certain things to suit your needs. First, it'll remove the empty calories you might have been eating throughout the snack time. Secondly, it'll train you to definitely stay away from unnecessary indulgences.

Switching towards the 16:8 Intermittent Fasting Routine

Once you happen to be at ease with lacking anything involving the meal, you should reduce the number of hours by which you have those meals. This means, you'll be able to still need three meals each day, but you should reduce the gap between breakfast and dinner. Suppose that you just previously had breakfast at 8 in the morning and dinner at 9 within the evening, this gives you simply 13-hour eating window. You should start implementing reducing this eating window. You can try shifting a single meal or both the meal a little bit. You might have your breakfast at 11 in the morning and dinner at 7 in the evening. This brings down your eating window to 8 hours. You can try any combination depending on your comfort. The only goal must be to minimize the eating window to 8 hours. This will give you a 16-hour fasting window. This needs to be the very first intermittent routine you follow. This routine is termed the 16:8 intermittent fasting routine.

It also offers you some weight loss benefits, and yes it is easy to follow.

You'll discover that you can follow this routine quite effortlessly. Let's examine the situation. An average person sleeps from 8-9 hours through the night. Doctors all around the globe unanimously advise people you can eat your last meal in the day 3-4 hours before going to sleep. Typically, you don't start eating once you get up. People have their breakfast 2-3 hours after they awaken. Even in case, you make small adjustments for a routine, following 16:8 intermittent fasting routine will be a cakewalk for you personally.

This can be a very powerful routine. It will give you most of the great things about intermittent fasting, and you wouldn't need to compromise on anything. In the 8-hour eating window, you can eat just about everything. This may be the first leg of intermittent fasting.

Important Fact

For those people that are attempting to rush this method, please take a minute. Your body is an efficient machine, but it still runs as being a machine. It has become running the body over a particular fuel, carbohydrates. Intermittent fasting is going to push your system to burn fat for fuel. Although fat is a cleaner and better fuel, your body isn't adapted to lose it inside the beginning. This is why a sluggish transition is extremely important. The means of losing weight is termed ketosis. Your body may take 3 days to 6 weeks to switch to ketosis and thus, rushing the process can prove to be counterproductive since it leaves you without any fuel in any respect throughout the transition.

Switching towards the 20:4 Intermittent Fasting Routine

Once you might be comfortable while using 16:8 fasting routine, only then should you move ahead. You should practice each method before you get accustomed to it. Never rush this process; your system should learn to sustain the limited method of getting blood glucose levels. Lack of this training will lead to 'Adrenaline Stress' in your system. You can start feeling light-headedness, tired, thirsty, weak, and many other similar problems. These are all hypoglycemic symptoms. This implies that the body suddenly goes to have less blood glucose. This can lead to irritability along with a strong hunger. It can be an undesirable condition. Earlier, frequent snacks and meals kept one's body furnished with blood glucose. It has caused great harm to one's body, but one's body has become used to it. Switching the routine prematurely is going to be equally harmful, which's why a pokey transition is suggested.

Once one's body gets used to the 16:8 intermittent fasting routine, you need to try narrowing your eating window again. Once you've assimilated for an 8-hour eating window, start decreasing that eating window by an hour or so. Meaning, it is possible to move to a 7-hour eating window. Once comfortable with that new fasting window, then take it down to 6, and so on.

At first, make an effort to eliminate one complete meal from a routine. You can make this happen by shifting your breakfast to the lunchtime. Bringing your eating window to 4 hours needs to be your main aim here.

In this, you'll fast for 20 hours and also have all your meals in the 4-hour eating window. As the eating window decreases, you'll believe it is difficult to eat three meals. Learning to own two healthy meals with this period is the best. You can consume the things you prefer within this window in a quantity. Intermittent fasting isn't a dieting routine. It is targeted on burning fat deposits stored in the body. Incidentally, after 20 hours of fasting, your capacity to eat food will decrease. You may feel completely hungry inside at the beginning; however, you wouldn't have the ability to nibble on food in a very plethora. The feeling of fullness will come quickly. This is really a challenging routine to which to adapt. Your body is going to take some time for you to get employed in this phase. However, this routine will return maximum weight reduction benefits.

The 4-hour eating window is really a minimal period. It is hard to get two full meals on this period, and you will probably end up with one fulfilling meal of the day.

This may be the One Meal a Day (OMAD) routine that ought to be your main goal.

The OMAD routine has good health and can help you burn fat fast and gain lean muscles. The popular misconception that you'll just become weak and lose muscles is flat wrong. The fact this is certainly one from the most popular methods in the bodybuilding community should clear your doubts. Bodybuilders heavily rely on this routine for shedding extra fat and gaining muscular mass.

Your body begins running on fat for fuel and become more effective and energetic. The OMAD routine will even bring extra benefits like autophagy, which can be an inside repair mechanism. The toxic waste in your system will probably be eliminated, and you will probably get additional benefits like increased growth and anti-aging too.

Boost the Benefits of OMAD Routine with Occasional Extended Water Fasting

Studies have repeatedly demonstrated the benefits of fasting. The important things about fasting far outweigh the efforts essential for fasting. It accelerates your fat loss efforts, cleanses, boosts anti-aging, and promotes longevity among other nutrients. Fasting gives our body to be able to recover and repair. If there is certainly one thing that offers an enhancement towards the effects of fasting, then it can be water fasting.

Water fasting, as the name suggests, is the entire process of keeping the short by only consuming water. You go without eating anything at all for longer periods. This kind of fasting can extend from 24 to 72 hours safely. People under supervision are able to keep water fasts after only longer and enjoy better health.

One thing is crucial to comprehend: you shouldn't undertake long water fasts without conferring with a physician. If you are afflicted by chronic illness, or you are on any medication, it will become every important. Water fasting is a serious business. It will bring about the appropriate cleansing and detoxification of your body system. Doing it without talking to a health care provider can cause complications for those on medication.

Water fasting, if done correctly, can do amazing things to your system. It revitalizes the whole system. One powerful process that takes over with water fasts is autophagy. This may be the internal repair and maintenance mechanism. Your body starts producing plenty of stem cells that result in the regeneration of lost cells and muscles.

Water fasting is a powerful tool that can give a head start for a healthy life. If you were already following an OMAD routine, then fasting won't be described as a problem in your case. Water fasting will cause relaxation of the gut.

Our whole body is a fancy mechanism. It works day-in and day-out tirelessly. However, one section of the body never gets rest, and that's your gut. It is actively working to digest food and replenish the nice gut bacteria. During water fasting, this method enjoys a much-needed respite. Therefore, as soon as the water fasting is over, your digestion mechanism improves considerably.

One critical thing that you must bear in mind while engaging in water fasting is that you simply shouldn't end your water fast inside a haphazard manner. The progression to eating must continually be slow and organized. Not doing this may be dangerous as your body takes time for you to adjust to the assault of food items.

You must plan carefully before and after the water fast. Your body is gonna cleanse itself during the water fast, and you must produce an environment to the.

Before a Water Fast

When you plan to begin your water fast, it is crucial that you go easy on food. Eating difficult-to-digest foods several days before water fast could be a bad idea. You will want your gut to unwind. Try to eat vegetable and fruit diets at the very least 3 days when you begin your water fast. These items are really easy to digest; also, your system is going to be in a position to clear them quickly. Meat and greasy food are tough to clean as it gets stuck, and thus consuming a great deal of meat and fatty foods will never be recommended.

During the Water Fast

Water fasting should continually be done on days when you are able to give your body time for it to relax. Weekends or long vacations are fantastic days for water fasts. Nowadays, your focus mustn't be on straining your system. You can give heavy exercise or strenuous activity an escape on these days. The first day ought to be easy as you will end up spending the force with the food consumed the day before. The second day will jump-start fat reducing because you will likely have less energy and your system will even start cleansing. Relaxing during this time is extremely helpful. On the next day, your system could have adapted on the fat loss, and you may glance at the surge of your energy. You may not be craving for any food in anyway. You can break your fast at the end of the third day with vegetable juice or broth.

Ending the Water Fast

Stopping the water fast can be a critical part. Your body may be in a relaxing mode. Your gut is clean and relaxed. If you commence eating whole grain products or hard vegetables around the first day of breaking your water fast, your gut may revolt. You will need to avoid that unpleasant scenario. Always end your water fast little by little. Start by drinking vegetable juice or broth because the first meal to interrupt your fast replenishes your whole body and doesn't strain it. Broth provides you with the nutrients and possesses less sugar. Therefore, there is often a very low risk of high blood sugar. You can also take vegetable soup later in the day to obtain energy. On the second day, you can eat fruit juice or smoothies too should you choose not to have problems like diabetes. You should begin slowly and take only soft or mashed food which is simple to digest. Give your gut time to adapt, and proceed to an excellent diet and raw vegetables slowly.

The progression is vital if you start out splurging soon after your water fast, then this whole effort falls to the drain.

Water fasting has immense benefits; however, it does put a little force on your body. Therefore, it can be essential to adopt all of the necessary precautions. If you do it correctly under supervision, this can provide you with great health benefits. The key to water fasting is control. If you have the habit of bingeing after fasts, then water fasting isn't for you.

Water fasting will cleanse your cells and result in weight loss. Your body can get enough time to obtain empty calories and get rid of fat reserves.

OMAD Routine and Keto Diet, a Match Made in Heaven

Overbearing fat is really a serious issue as well as a reality in the current American lifestyle. With the majority of the American population facing the obesity epidemic, we cannot keep feigning ignorance. The OMAD routine presents a straightforward strategy to lose fat. It is sustainable and intensely effective. You will not just lose the temporary water weight but in addition, actually burn the visceral fat once and for all.

A Ketogenic diet makes it possible to achieve. The Keto diet is the right way to lose weight. For beginners, the ketogenic diet is a high-fat, moderate protein, and low-carbohydrate diet. It shifts one's body from burning carbohydrates to fat.

For those people who find themselves wondering, once they adopt an OMAD routine burning extra fat, how come they keep consuming more fat? There is definitely an answer. However, for you, you are going to need to see the mechanism through which your body uses energy.

We usually run our own bodies on carbohydrate fuel. Most of the things we eat are an excellent source of carbohydrates. It is digested quickly and gives us glucose. Our liver can process it quicker than our pancreas releases insulin to use up everything that glucose. The extra glucose then gets transformed into glycogen and fat. However, within this whole process, our body is only using carbohydrates and stops losing fat. This creates the entire problem of fat accumulation inside the first place.

When you start a keto diet, you deprive the body of carbohydrate fuel and force it to burn off fat. The fat is a difficult fuel to burn but releases a higher amount of ounce. In this method, our body also starts burning its excess fat to power itself, after which real fat reduction occurs.

However, our own bodies will not start losing fat until and unless the method of getting carbohydrate fuel turned off. Two very different sorts of mechanisms are required for burning these energy sources. Eventually, insulin is in the base of the whole problem.

When you happen to be continuously eating high carbohydrate and abusing your system with frequent meals, insulin resistance begins.

You start facing a multiple of problems like:

·Belly Fat

·Hypertension

·Diabetes

·Fatigue

·Memory loss

·Lack of focus

·Anxiety

·Depression

Your body stops addressing high insulin secretion and develops insulin resistance. We have already discussed that insulin resistance results in problems and excess weight are certainly one included in this.

One way to have excess insulin resistance and increase insulin sensitivity would be to lower blood glucose levels. This is what the keto diet does to suit your needs.

When you go on the keto diet within your OMAD routine, your blood sugar levels go down, and your system switches to burning fat deposits fuel set up of carbohydrate fuel. Lowering sugar intake is often a critical requirement for this technique to start.

You can certainly satisfy this disorder by switching to some keto diet. However, there may be some initial difficulties using this type of process. Your body may be hooked on sugar. When you set about a low-carbohydrate diet, your blood sugar levels may drop.

You may face the next symptoms within a few days:

·Strong cravings

·Lightheadedness

·Hunger

·Fatigue

·Constipation

You won't have to worry a lot of about these symptoms as they are temporary and they're going to recede as time passes. There are easy ways to manage these symptoms.

You can ward off the original problems by doing the next things:

Fatigue: B5 deficiency. You may feel fatigue within the beginning. You can certainly overcome this fatigue if you take Vitamin B5 supplements.

Cramps: Potassium deficiency. Cramps and constipation is a common issue. However, most of the problem is as a result of potassium deficiency, and you are able to overcome it by consuming vegetables. While you might be over a keto diet, have a lot of greens. Cruciferous vegetables have lots of potassium, and they will support these symptoms. They are incredibly healthy and fulfill a vitamin and mineral deficiency.

Bloating: Bile Salts. Bloating is also a very common problem encountered by people with a keto diet. An easy approach to deal with this issue is to consume foods low in fats. People will start consuming a lot of fat on the start. Understand that one's body is going to create a switch. You will need to go slow for the fat. Take sea salt set up of table salt and increase its daily intake a little. This will help you in overcoming the problems.

Sleep Issues: Calcium Magnesium deficiency. People start facing problems associated with sleep. This can easily be managed by consuming lots of green vegetables. They contain a great deal of calcium and magnesium, as well as your sleep would improve.

Decalcification: Take Lime. The keto diet, as well as the OMAD routine results in decalcification. Many calcium deposits which can be clogging one's body get cleaned. This may cause the introduction of urates and kidney stones. The easy approach to manage this problem would be to improve the intake of lemon. Consume at the very least one lemon in a day or more. Drink fresh limewater or lemon or citrus fruits, but consuming lemon is important. This will help in cleaning one's body and allow you to avoid these complaints.

One more problem people face while around the keto diet, and also the OMAD routine is that they feel too stuffed. The reason behind this issue is overeating. You possess a fewer number of meals every day. You attempt to eat around as you can. Although there's no calorie restriction inside OMAD routine, overeating will make you feel stuffed. Do not overeat. Your body will run fine on fat inside lack of calorie intake.

Some people find that their cholesterol levels increase while on a keto diet. There is no reason to have alarmed. This cholesterol is not dietary cholesterol. When your system burns fat, it releases cholesterol and triglycerides. It uses them as fuel and for that reason;

the amount can be naturally higher in comparison with a typical state. However, cholesterol is just not a dangerous thing. It could be the source of hormones along with other beneficial things in your system. Your levels of cholesterol will stabilize as time passes, so you would start feeling great.

The important things would be to get off sugar. As long as you have easily available glucose fuel, even just in small quantities, your system won't start burning fat. Your body takes around 72 hours to use all the accessible energy stored available as glucose and glycogen. Once these sources are depleted, your body doesn't have other option rather than burn up fat. You will not simply lose water weight with all the help of the keto diet but may also lose fat around your belly. This implies that for a length, your waist circumference will shrink and you will probably use a leaner body.

Some people believe that from a certain period they stop losing weight with a keto diet. There is really a strong reason for yours. Once your body loses the lake weight and starts losing fat, your body also starts building muscular mass. Muscle is dense, more than fat. So you get thinner, while your weight may increase. This is an advantage. The correct strategy to measure your progress on the keto weight loss program is to measure unwanted weight in addition to waist circumference. Your weight may stop decreasing after having a certain length of time; however, your waist circumference can keep shrinking.

The keto diet makes it possible to lose fat and get a leaner and muscular frame. You become healthy and still have an abundance of their time. You will feel good all day and get going to many lifestyle disorders.

There are seven strong important things about using a Keto Diet:

High Energy Levels. Fat fuel may be the superior fuel for your body. It leaves no toxic waste and keeps the body running for long, that's why one's body chooses to store it for contingency measures. This fuel can make you stay running healthily for long even on the smaller diet.

Weight Loss. The keto diet accelerates your fat loss. This diet blocks your carbohydrate intake. You start running your body on fat. This helps to burn unwanted fat. You will reduce weight quickly and get a much better figure. It is the greatest way to gain lean muscular mass.

Improved Memory. The keto diet offers you a huge amount of antioxidants. They help together with your brain function. The alteration in hormones also improves in the body which helps in neurological function. The OMAD routine along which has a keto diet gives an enhancement to autophagy that improves memory and decreases neurodegenerative disorders.

Improves Mood. The fluctuating glucose levels with a carbohydrate meal can provide you with mood swings.

This just isn't the truth with all the fat fuel. The fat fuel burns slowly but consistently and releases an increased amount of ounce. This keeps your mood stable, and you also stop experiencing moodiness.

Cravings and Hunger Go Away. This is one of the best advantages of being on the Keto diet while following an OMAD routine. As your body keto-adapts, it stops having the cravings for sugar and hunger pangs. It has a steady source of energy, and you do not feel hunger for very long. The people on longer fasts stop feeling hunger. Therefore, you'll be able to have a great focus, plus your attention will probably be undivided.

Better Metabolism. The keto diet improves your metabolism. Your body burns fat more efficiently and yields excellent results.

Improves Insulin Resistance. Insulin may be described as a reason for most of the health problems, but it can be a necessary hormone. Insulin resistance caused by disorderly food consumption can cause several problems. The OMAD routine along with a keto diet helps you in improving insulin dysfunction and restore insulin sensitivity. It is highly beneficial for you personally and may bring positive health effects.

Important Things To Remember With The One Meal A Day Diet

Whenever you are trying anything new or different or radically alter your lifestyle, try not to get too difficult on yourself if things don't go as smoothly as you hoped. It happens. That's life. It's important to remember that slip-ups can happen. If you can't make an immediate change, that's okay. You can begin by eating three smaller meals a day and gradually restricting till you might be at one meal, or have healthy, low-calorie snacks like fruit if you are able to make it to your designated meal time in the beginning.

Don't worry if the body weight doesn't instantly go. You'll notice five to ten points go straight away. Most people do. That's your water weight. Your body flushes it out of your body system in the event its given time to fast. After that, it might be a few months before you see any significant change inside your weight. Make sure that you do not eat foods high in sodium simply because they make you retain water. Don't stuff yourself. Only eat until you're satisfied.

Don't under eat with the intention of slimming down faster. This isn't a starvation diet! It's a way to take your mind away from food, let you live your health, reach your ideal weight range, and appreciate food more whenever you do eat. If you under eat, you'll only achieve short term as opposed to long lasting weight reduction.

It's okay to nibble on more or more often during holidays, vacations, or special attractions. Having "splurge days" is a component with the plan. Enjoy yourself at Thanksgiving, Christmas, or New Year's but get back on track the following day. One Meal a Day isn't about restrictions but the variety and freedom to eat what you want and still lose fat. Enjoy yourself. That's part of life too.

Conclusion

Change is hard, but change can also be worth some time and effort you add put to it. You also should remember to become realistic. Results won't happen overnight, but they will happen. One meal each day is amongst one of the most natural ways to nibble on. Our ancestors ate less often and didn't have any problems with obesity or many of the medical problems we face in the world today. Thanks to constant access to food - both good and bad - people don't appreciate the quality, texture, and flavor of food all them anymore. Our ancestors were healthy, happy, and appreciated food. You can bring that back by pursuing the One Meal a Day Diet.

PART 2

Objection!!!

I've heard it all! You'll get ulcer. You're starving yourself. You're destroying your body. You're an idiot. You don't know what you're doing. You don't know anything. You don't need to lose weight. The doctor says... This expert said... I read online... I saw on YouTube... I read a research (which usually they skimmed through and didn't understand)... You don't go hungry? Why!? That's torture! Can't you afford food? Life is short. You're not enjoying life. You must be miserable. On and on and on... I get those remarks from friends, family, loved ones, strangers, colleagues, and experts.

Some people say I'm lean because I'm Asian. Not true. You might've missed the headlines but China has the largest number of obese children in the world.[8] Health or lack of it is not a white, black, or latino thing. It affects Asians as much as other races. Actually, Asians, it seems, are more susceptible to diabetes and have a lower rate of fat metabolism compared to caucasians.[9]

Despite the naysayers, I think I'm doing something right. I look younger. I'm fit and I'm strong. I may not be a supermodel or Mr. Olympia but I think I look good. You'll be the judge when you visit my Instagram profile. The naysayers are either fat, flabby, weak, and/or have health problems. I have none to date. So I think I'm on the right track.

I have been eating a meal a day for years. If there's a problem it would've shown by now. I only went to the hospital twice in my adult life. First was when I was in Haiti, I got pneumonia. The second was in the Philippines when I got a piece of drywall in my eyes which caused corneal abrasion. If you took "went to the hospital" literally, then yes, I went more than twice to visit sick people who eat all the time. Suffice it to say, OMAD didn't cause my hospital visits.

It's true you won't get big Mr. Olympia muscles eating one meal a day. If you're bodybuilding or if you have high-energy requirements OMAD may not be a good idea, unless if you could cram all the calories you need and more in one meal. Women should be very careful of food deprivation. A woman's body reacts differently to food deprivation than men. Some women miss their period when they don't consume enough calories.

The consensus is never eat less than 1,200 calories per day for safe weight loss. For those who want to lose weight safely, various sources recommend cutting 250-500 calories per day. Never treat OMAD as a crash diet. It will backfire. Don't go OMAD then not meet your nutritional requirements just to cut calories. It could only go horribly wrong. Most people who experience adverse effects on calorie restriction is because of bad nutrition.

Be warned, people on OMAD may have some "abnormalities" in their blood work, especially when the checkup is done in the morning. My most recent test results are as follows:

TEST NAME	MY RESULT	NORMAL
Glucose (sugar)	104.1 mg/dL	70-105 mg/dL
LDL Cholesterol "Bad" Cholesterol	145.2 mg/dL	65-150 mg/dL
HDL Cholesterol "Good" Cholesterol	72.9 mg/dL	45 mg/dl
Triglycerides	76 mg/dL	150 mg/dL
Cholesterol	203 mg/dL	0-200 mg/dL

My doctor was primarily concerned with my blood glucose and my cholesterol since diabetes and cardiovascular diseases run in the family. But since I'm healthy and exercise regularly, his concerns were abated. My results, though high, still falls within the normal range. Cholesterol is slightly high by 3 mg/dl but since my triglycerides are low and my HDL or the "good" cholesterol is high, my doctor was appeased.

I don't know how relevant this is to my blood test but in the interest of being thorough, these tests were done while I was traveling. I had a transpacific flight. The combination of jet lag, lack of sleep, and general stress of traveling long distances might've affected the results. Stress can increase blood sugar levels and LDL cholesterol levels.

I'm not worried. There's a logical explanation for this.

You'll Have Ulcer!

"Doc, I eat one meal a day. I exercise 3-4 times a week, sometimes 5. I don't smoke. I don't do drugs. I drink only on rare occasions. I eat plenty of vegetables and avoid processed food." I said. "One meal a day? How are you feeling." He asked. "Uh, normal?" He gave me an appraising look and said, "No stomach aches?" He asked. "None. Why?" I replied. "I'm just concerned with peptic ulcers. There's no food to neutralize your stomach acids." My doctor explained in a matter of fact way. "But doc, peptic ulcer is caused by bacteria or stress. No?"

Until the 80s people believed ulcer is caused by excessive stomach acid secretion or certain foods. This, however, is not true. The most common cause of peptic ulcer is a bacteria called Helicobacter pylori, identified in 1982 by Australian scientists Barry Marshall and Robin Warren.[10]

People taking NSAIDs (Nonsteroidal Anti-Inflamatory Drugs) and aspirin are four times likely to get ulcers than non-users. Although stress was ruled out as cause of ulcer, stress together with other risk factors may increase risk of ulcers due to the effects of stress on gastric physiology.[11]

Eating one meal a day will not cause your stomach acids to poke holes through your stomach. I've never had any stomach aches, hyperacidity, acid reflux, let alone ulcers on OMAD. Not even during 3-4 days of fasting.

Your stomach is perfectly capable of handling the acid it produces. Acid production in the stomach decreases when you don't eat, it's why after very long fasts it's recommended reintroducing food slowly. It's evolutionarily dumb to have an organ constantly produce a substance which destroys it.

Your High Blood Sugar

"Your uncles died of diabetes. I'm concerned about your blood sugar." My doctor said. "I don't even eat sugar and I eat few simple carbs. No junk food as well." I replied. "You're within normal range but you're borderline." He was referring to my high blood sugar. "Do I get Metformin now? Please?" I said, exploiting the chance to get a prescription drug for diabetes which according to research may slow aging. "Why?" My doctor asked incredulously. "Because blood sugar." I said. "You don't need it. We would have to do further tests if you're really concerned with diabetes. I can't just diagnose you with diabetes based on one blood test." Apparently, one blood test is not enough for him to prescribe me a diabetes drug. Sigh.

Your body uses glucose (sugar) as a source of energy. A hormone produced by your pancreas called insulin moves glucose from your bloodstream into your cells so they can be used as energy. When you sleep your body uses less energy but when you're about to wake up, your body will need more fuel—more sugar.[12]

The dawn effect or the dawn phenomenon is the rise in blood sugar released by the liver as a person's body prepares to wake up from sleep.[13] *Every person* experiences the dawn phenomenon.[14]

The Somogyi effect may also explain rise in blood sugar for people on OMAD. It was first described by Michael Somogyi as the body defenses responding to long periods of low blood sugar such as when a person exercises a lot, takes more insulin than needed before bed, or goes a long time without snack.[15] I.e. eats one meal a day or fasts.

This explains the "abnormal" increase in blood sugar for those on OMAD. Your body has to manufacture its own fuel somehow.

It's like a one-two punch. Based on the dawn and Somogyi effects, we'll really experience an upshot in blood sugar, especially in the morning. We're going for long periods of time (at least 20 hours) without food and our body needs sugar to wake up.

I take this rise in sugar in my blood stream as my body making breakfast.

I don't remember which experts said this but in essence what causes insulin resistance and diabetes is insulin. They explained, the body gets used to stimuli. You need more and more of the same stimuli to achieve the same effect. For example if you drink alcohol, over time you develop a tolerance for alcohol and need more and more quantity to get drunk. The same is true with insulin resistance. When you repeatedly spike up your insulin level like when you eat simple carbohydrates (e.g. sugars), your body will develop tolerance to the high levels of insulin. Over time, you'll need more and more insulin to have the same effect. Eventually, your body will develop insulin resistance or diabetes.

These are the reason why I'm not concerned with diabetes. In addition, one blood sugar test won't determine if I'm diabetic. Multiple tests are needed to diagnose diabetes. But if you're concerned regarding your blood sugar level or diabetes, consult your doctor.

Your High Cholesterol

"Your LDL, bad cholesterol, is high. Within normal but high." He looked at the chart again. "Your cholesterol is borderline. 3 mg/dl more than where I want it to be." I know why he's so concerned. My father recently died of stroke. My aunts and uncles have cholesterol problems. He looked up from the chart as I curled my arm showing my bicep and lifted my shirt to show my toned abs. "Does this look fat and unhealthy?" My doctor and his assistant laughed. "You're healthy. Your HDL, the good cholesterol is high. It must be tipping the cholesterol ratio. Your triglycerides are also low. You just need to watch it though. Your dad died of stroke and I'm concerned about your cholesterol level."

Let's discuss cholesterol in more detail because we'll go back to it in our later discussions.

I eat a lot of fats. I'm personally not worried about cholesterol and LDL levels (Low Density Lipoproteins, what's considered "bad" cholesterol). Besides my HDL is high (High Density Lipoproteins, what's considered "good") and my triglycerides are low. Translation: the standard good markers are high and the standard bad markers are low or within normal range.

If I don't eat during the day, my body has to break down fats and dump it in my blood to deliver fuel to every cell, tissue, and organ in my body. Naturally, cholesterol level has to then go up. This was reflected by my test results. This is my body making it's own food.

The "cholesterol and saturated fats are bad for you" dictum is a myth. According to Nina Teicholz, author of New York Times bestseller The Big Fat Surprise: Why Butter, Meat and Cheese Belong in a Healthy Diet, changing your LDL cholesterol levels through diet has no effect on your cardio vascular outcomes.[16]

You also need to ask yourself, if cholesterol is so bad, why does our body produce it? Your brain is made of 20% cholesterol.[17] Steroid hormones like Testosterone and Estrogen come from cholesterol.[18] Your cell walls are made up of cholesterol.[19] Your nerves are lined with cholesterol. Cholesterol is what allows communication and electrical exchange between nerve cells.[20] There's no healthy brain without cholesterol. Period. Cholesterol is essential to life. So why is cholesterol bad? It's all over your body and it's performing vital functions. Your body even produces it when supplies are low.

The myth and our fear of saturated fats began back in the 50s with the Diet-Heart Hypothesis. Ancel Keys' Seven Countries Study concluded saturated fats cause cardiovascular diseases and eating less saturated fats lead to less cardiovascular diseases.[21] I'm paraphrasing of course. With this conclusion our fear of fats began. We started obsessing with LDL and cholesterol counts. Low fat diet became the norm and cholesterol-lowering drugs were prescribed left and right. We've been at war against fats since then. But Ancel Keys was wrong. So wrong.

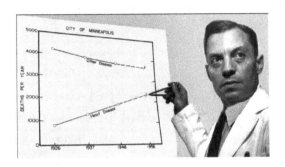

Ancel Keys, the man who got the world scared of cholesterol. Photo: modally.com

Keys' study clearly showed a correlation between saturated fats and heart disease. As saturated fat intake increased, heart disease increased in the 7 countries which were included in the study. What was wrong with his study you ask? There were 22 countries for which data was available, not seven![22] Countries like Denmark, France, Norway have a high fat intake but has low occurrence of heart disease. Countries like Chile has low fat intake but high in occurrence of heart disease. When such countries are factored in, the correlation is not so clear anymore.[23] In fact, they called this data discrepancy a paradox, coined in the term the "French Paradox"–the source of the ad hoc idea red wine is good for you.

Since when do you call data which doesn't fit your conclusion a paradox? If the data doesn't match your conclusion then there's something wrong with your conclusion. Clearly there's something wrong with Keys' theory.

The next problem with Keys' study is it's an observational study. It establishes correlation but not causation. There was no double blind studies or trials of any sort. He saw increased heart disease and increased saturated fat intake in 7 countries, presto! Saturated fat is the cause of heart disease. Think of Keys' correlation like this: There are always firemen when houses are on fire. Therefore, firemen cause fires.

When scientists looked at the data in 2010, the connection between saturated fats and heart diseases isn't so strong anymore. A meta-analysis (a study of other studies) concluded: *"There was no significant evidence that saturated fat is associated with an increased risk of cardiovascular disease."* This was also echoed by the Annals of Internal Medicine's meta-analysis involving 80 studies and more than half a million subjects. A team in Cambridge University led by a cardiovascular epidemiologist Dr. Rajiv Chowdhury concluded: *"The evidence does not support low consumption of saturated fats or high consumption of polyunsaturated fats are considered heart healthy.*"[24]

In other words, the Seven Countries Study is not replicable. Put differently, all the experts who told you fats are bad for you were wrong. Put another way, you can eat butter and not clog your arteries.

The idea of dietary cholesterol as the major culprit of heart disease was dropped in 2013 by the American Heart Association.[25] The rest of the world hasn't caught up yet. At the time of this writing the average person still fears cholesterol like the plague. Many doctors still think fats are bad for you.

Your Lowered Mojo

"Doc, my testosterone levels are very very low!" I was looking at a chart which indicates: Normal. But it's on the lower end! I don't like this result! I want high testosterone! High! I'm a man for crying out loud! "Angie, does this look low to you?" My doctor's assistant looked at my chart and said, "It's good. Normal." She shrugged. "Doc, you need to prescribe me testosterone." I looked at my doctor, "I need testosterone!" I suddenly felt like a drug addict asking for Morphine as doc's assistant gave me an appraising look. I relented. "Ok. Doc. What do I do to raise my testosterone?" I said slightly defeated. "Eat oily fish like salmon. You need Omega 3 fatty acids. You can supplement with beta-alanine if you want."

Although OMAD definitely doesn't make men impotent and doesn't necessarily lead to menstrual problems in women, in my experience there's a palpable decrease in sex drive after a few months of eating one meal a day. It must be I'm in the age. It may also be because of catabolism, the break down of molecules in the body for energy. In a catabolic state, testosterone drops reducing sex drive.

There are anecdotes which suggests caloric restriction affects women differently than men. Women it seems are more sensitive to calorie restriction and can affect a woman's menstrual cycles.[26] I'm not a woman so I won't pretend to understand what women go through. However, I can deduce why our reproductive system and sexual drives are affected by OMAD.

To be clear, I said I had *decreased* sex drive, not zero sex drive. I don't have problems performing for my lover. I just noticed I wasn't as sexually driven as I was before. People on IF reported the same. This happens because fasting and reproduction have opposing goals.

When fasting your body is focused on self-preservation. It needs to save energy for important bodily functions until you can find food. Looking at it from evolution's point of view, decreased sexual drive makes sense. When food is scarce, there's very little sense in making babies.

As I've said earlier, OMAD is not for everybody. If you're pregnant, trying to get pregnant, or nursing, maybe it's not a good idea to eat one meal per day. Again, consult your doctor and maybe do some tests.

A lot of the anecdotes I read online about people losing their sex drive and women missing their periods came from people practicing IF improperly. I noticed, a lot of these people jump into the IF bandwagon abruptly. Their body simply doesn't have time to adapt to the new regimen. In this book I recommend gradually reducing food quantity before removing anything from your diet to avoid any possible issues. It took me over a year to fully go OMAD. It's a slow process. Most treat IF like crash diets not as a sensible eating habit.

Another reason for this negative effect may be macronutrient and calorie deficits. Some people simply focus on losing weight (nothing wrong with it), instead of focusing on being healthy. If you're centered on just losing weight, it's easy not to eat enough to meet dietary needs. Even if you're eating one meal a day, it's still important to meet dietary requirements. The expert consensus of safe caloric deficit for weight loss ranges from 250-500 calories per day and not consume less than 1,200 calories a day. I bet most people are cutting more and not eating the minimum in addition to missing important macronutrients.

Severe caloric deficits have serious consequences, especially for women's reproductive system. In a study in Germany, 31% of raw foodists indicated chronic caloric deficiency. In women it disrupted their menstrual cycle.[27]

Another culprit may be lack of protein, a macronutrient deficiency. Women preferred plant-based food and consumed less meat than men.[28] I would assume women on IF consumed even less meat. Protein is very important because your body is made up of proteins and protein is needed to repair every tissue in the body.

Women are more drawn to plant-based foods[29] which contain fewer calories and less proteins compared to meat. If you don't eat enough to meet caloric requirements and you don't have enough protein to prevent tissue loss, it's easy to think where stories of women missing their period while on IF comes from.

During the editing of this book, my editor told me women can also miss their periods due to sudden lifestyle changes. She personally experienced this after traveling for a few days. The effect lasted for months.

This is why when women miss their menstrual cycles doctors usually ask (other than recent sexual activity) if women travelled, got sick, or made any abrupt life changes.

You're Definitely Not Starving

You're starving yourself! a friend protested when I told her I eat one meal a day for health. I might intermittently be hungry on OMAD when I first started but I'm far from starving myself. Let's straighten this out. Starvation is not hunger.

Starvation is a dangerous medical condition which could lead to death characterized by a severe deficiency in caloric intake below the level needed to maintain an organism's life.[30] You can survive for 3-7 days without water[31] and 30-40 days without food. Symptoms of starvation don't appear until 35-40 days[32] not within a few hours after breakfast.

Hunger is a sensation, a motivational state, which represents the physiological need for food.[33] Sure, hunger is really unpleasant but hunger is neither fatal nor deadly. Eating one meal a day may cause you to feel hungry but it's neither dangerous nor deadly.

A lot of people confuse starvation and hunger because most people, especially in the developed worlds, rarely go without food for more than 6 hours.

After eating, the sugars from your meal stay for 5-6 hours before your blood sugar goes back to normal.[34] That is usually the time it takes for you to go from breakfast to lunch. It takes 12-22 hours, depending on

76

your activity, for your body to deplete its glycogen stores[35] (stored sugars) which an average person will likely never will.

What people call hunger is likely a sugar slump (usually characterized by lethargy, crankiness, and inability to concentrate) experienced after the high of eating carbohydrates.

The Sugar Trap

If you eat sugar your body will inevitably have to produce insulin. If you remember from the previous chapter, insulin is a hormone which drives sugars into your cells. When you eat, the sugars from your meal go to your blood stream. Blood sugar rises. Your body senses this rise in blood sugar, your pancreas release insulin to move the glucose (sugar in the body) in your blood into your cells where it can be used for energy.

The problem is, insulin is antagonistic (it inhibits) hormone-sensitive lipase (HSL), a hormone which mobilizes your fats for energy.[36] This means, if you keep eating meals with sugars (and when I say sugars I don't only mean the white stuff, I mean all carbohydrates like bread, rice, and pasta etc.) you won't use fats for energy because the insulin in your blood prevents hormone-sensitive lipase from doing its job. You won't use up stored glycogen (stored sugar) in your liver and skeletal muscles either because sugar is readily available from the meal you just ate. This creates a vicious cycle. I call it the sugar trap. It's why people feel three meals a day very necessary.

• You're hungry. You eat.

• You eat. Insulin is released to drive sugar into your cells for energy.

• Blood sugar drops in a few hours. You get cranky, lethargic, and low in energy. You interpret this as hunger.

• Insulin still lingers in your blood stream,[37] HSL can't mobilize fats for energy.

• You eat and start the cycle all over again.

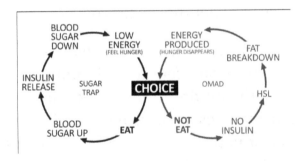

Every time you're hungry you have a choice to eat or not to eat. Every time you eat you release insulin and use glucose for energy. Every time you don't eat you go through your glycogen stores then breakdown fat stores. Technically, you can continue denying hunger... until, of course, you run out of energy and die of starvation. But we won't do it. We're in OMAD not a hunger strike. Just be mindful of the sugar trap.

In my experience, eating one meal a day makes you less hungry not more. This is echoed by what we know about Ghrelin—the hunger hormone. Ghrelin makes you feel hungry.

Hunger has a learned component.[38] Rise in Ghrelin coincides with people's meal times. In other words, you teach your body to be hungry all the time by eating three meals a day.

Hunger doesn't progressively become worst as time passes. In people who fast, Ghrelin levels are stable. People are no more or less hungry than when they started.[39] I have the same experience. I don't get progressively hungrier the longer I delay eating.

Hunger wanes. If you could hold off eating it disappears. You won't feel it again until it reappears later. The more you do it the less you feel hunger as mealtime approaches. In my experience fasting, hunger doesn't appear until 24-48 hours of my last meal. It's at its worst on the second or third day. Later we'll discuss specific strategies to deal with hunger and how to reduce food consumption to make the transition from three to one meal easier.

One Meal A Day Benefits

Eating One Meal A Day

I couldn't believe it! Six to eight meals cost a lot! I'm literally spending a small fortune on food. While agonizing on my expenses YouTube tugged on one of my ears. It was one of the videos on life extension I was watching. "Are there any life prolonging techniques that actually work today?" It started with a question, the exact question constantly on my mind. "There is one." It continued while showing an image of a yeast cell. "...if you feed yeast cells less, they live longer. So do nematode worms. Fruit flies and even rodents." The video got my full attention now. "It seems that semi-starvation extends lifespan." There it was, the answer to reducing my expenses and living longer. This was the solution I was looking for!

If you want to lose weight, be healthier, have more time during the day, and have more money in your pocket, you literally have to do one thing: eat one meal a day. It doesn't matter how big the meal is. Eat whatever and as much as you want. We're aiming for a period of food deprivation then a period of relative indulgence.

When I say one meal a day (OMAD) I mean a full course meal–appetizers, main course, dessert. We eat until we're full then we stop. You can go for second or third servings if one is not enough. I want to stress: eat whatever and as much quantity as you want. Don't worry about overeating, your body won't allow you to. Unless of course you behave like a professional eater. I know I said you can eat whatever you want, but be reasonable with this. If you know something is bad for you don't eat it. The aim is to consume nothing except water for the day, then eat as much as you want in the evening or afternoon.

I know it sounds crazy. Even extreme for some but it's neither crazy nor extreme. I would argue, this should be the norm especially in an era when people sit still more than they move. If it worked for ancient warriors on the move, it would definitely work for desk-bound warriors of today.[40]

Eating one meal a day has a lot of benefits.[41] Those benefits include:

1. Weight loss

2. Lowered risk of diabetes

3. Improved blood sugar control

4. Improved cardiovascular health

5. Improved brain health

6. Reduced inflammation

7. Reduced risk of cancer

8. Live longer

9. Stable energy level

10. Less hunger and cravings

I know these are subjective but some immediate benefits of OMAD I experienced include:

1. Better focus

2. Better sleep

3. Sharper senses

4. Looking younger

5. Having a better body

6. More time during the day

7. More money saved at the end of the month

8. Simplification of life.

To date, I have not experienced any adverse effects on OMAD. But I would be committing a lie of omission if I don't say there are people who probably should not eat one meal a day. Those people are pregnant or nursing women, children, growing teens, malnourished people, and bodybuilders who want to gain weight. People with high energy requirements like athletes and marathon runners, and people who have psychological problems related to food should not eat one meal a day.

Eating one meal a day is not a quick fix solution or something you try for a specified period of time just to lose weight fast. It may backfire on you. This is not a fad diet. OMAD only works if it becomes your routine.

Lose Weight

Ahhh, the magic word in everyone's fat minds. Lose weight. It doesn't matter whether you're in North America, Europe, or Asia. The world is getting fat according to worldwide trends. If you're overweight or obese, losing weight should be your priority. If not, maintaining your weight is a must. Carrying excess amount of fats is associated with all sorts of bad health outcomes.

Whether you eat or not, your body has to find a way to constantly supply itself with energy, even at sleep. If it doesn't you die. If you're not eating, your body doesn't have a ready supply of energy from food. So it has to breakdown stored glycogen and fats for energy. As a result, you lose weight.

When you eat, blood sugar rises. Fat burning stops and you start using glucose from the food you just ate for energy. When you stop burning fats you stop losing weight. Glucose you don't use for energy replenishes glycogen stores, then whatever is left is converted into fats. In other words, you gain weight. If there are not enough fat cells to store the converted fats, your body makes more fat cells. You become fat, overweight, or obese if you keep this up.

Eating (especially carbohydrates) stimulates the release of insulin which in turn signals storage of food energy. Not eating stimulates Glucagon and hormone-sensitive lipase which in turn signals the breakdown of stored food energy, i.e. fats.

It sounds like a joke but it's true, if you want to lose weight, *don't eat*.

Unfortunately, if you don't want to lose weight on OMAD the best you can do is minimize weight loss until your weight stabilizes. Losing weight is simply the side effect of breaking down fats for energy. You can increase or decrease food intake depending on your target weight.

I was 85 kg. (187 lbs.) going to 90 kg. (200 lbs.) when I was eating 8-6 meals for body building. I was 75 kg. (165 lbs.) when I cut down to eating three meals a day. In a few months of OMAD I dropped to 65 kg. (143 lbs), then settled around there—I did everything I can not to lose weight. At the time of this writing, my weight still remains at a 60-65 kg (132-143 lbs) range. Sometimes a bit more, sometimes a bit less but nothing drastic.

Rest assured your weight will stabilize at a certain range. Your body doesn't want to consume muscle tissue essential for bodily functions when there's fat to burn.[42] As a result your weight is maintained at a specific range.

For those who want to maintain weight, an average man should consume the recommended 3,000-3,500 calories per day while an average woman should consume 2,000-2,500 calories per day. Even then, in my experience, you'll lose weight. Unfortunately. Having a period of food deprivation like what we have in OMAD is so effective at burning fats, making you lose weight.

I've given up tracking my weight on the scale. Instead, I use a mirror. If I like what I see I continue doing what I'm doing. If not, I modify what I'm doing. I also take reference photos of myself to compare. What I see is a better gauge. Nobody walks around with a scale but everybody has eyes. People judge what they see not some abstract number.

More Time

As a bodybuilder in the past, I ate 8 times a day. Breakfast, snack, lunch, snack, pre-wrokout snack, post-workout snack, dinner, snack/dessert. I ate all the time yet I always felt hungry. It was a lot. I was painfully aware of how much time it takes to acquire, prepare, and consume food.

Food-related activities simply take too much time. If you could cut down time spent acquiring, making, and consuming food, you gain more time during the day. Time after all is finite and unrenewable.

You have 24 hours in a day. You spend at least 20 hours sleeping, commuting, and working. If you allocate three hours for three meals a day you've already spent 23 hours. Then you have to go to the toilet... what's left of your time?

I gained so much time for other activities just by eating one meal a day. I don't have to spend too much time eating and I reduced the time needed for food-related activities. I cook once a week for 1.5-2 hours instead of cooking an hour every day. It's called batch processing. I store the food in the fridge and reheat my meals when I'm ready to eat. I consume my one meal in an hour or less because the less time I spend with food the more time I have to do other things. The exception is when I eat in social gatherings or when I eat with another person, then I spend more time on my meal.

Not having precooked meals creates an opportunity for eating out or eating processed foods. Having food already prepared for the week ensures I have good food ready to eat. There's no excuse to eat processed food or dubious takeout food.

You can cook everyday to make your single meal special but it just burns more time. With a busy life, do you have time to cook fresh food everyday? Most people assume they have time to prepare and cook food but with 20 hours already burned for daily activities, do you really want to spend your remaining hours cooking? It's more time efficient to batch process cooking than to cook every time you need to eat.

More Money

Food is one of the biggest item in a household's budget.[43] In the US, in 2017, middle income households spent 14.3% of income on food, while lower income households spent 34.1% of income on food.[44]

I used to spend on average $150 per week on groceries and food-related expenses (I used to live in Haiti where food costs an arm and a leg and a first-born male child). In a month it's $600 or $7,200 per year–I can go on a month vacation to Paris with that money!

Eating one meal a day reduced my groceries and food-related expenses in Haiti by a third. On average I was spending $50 a week on food. $75 max on some occasions.

Let's do the math. $50 per week is $200 in a month and $2,400 in a year. By eating one meal per day I'm saving $4,800 annually. It's a substantial reduction in my living expenses and I only have to literally do one thing: OMAD. Not to mention I'm gaining time which is very hard to put a fix value on.

The thinking is to maximize economic potential. By saving money I could invest more. By gaining back time I could make more money. More time means more opportunities to do other things.

Those are just the immediate financial benefits of OMAD. In the long term, imagine the money you'll save on medication and doctor fees. Healthcare is expensive.

It's an odd thing. I see people trading away health and neglecting their body to make money only to spend all their money trying to regain the health they've squandered and will never get back. The healthier you are the less money you need to spend on healthcare thus saving you money in the longterm.

Put like this, eating one meal a day becomes a very easy decision to make. It's a no brainer!

More Energy

It's not that you have more energy when you eat one meal a day, you're just allowing your body to tap into its energy stores which contain more energy than a single meal. Using an internal source of fuel (fats) results in stable energy levels which makes you feel as if you have more energy because you don't feel energy slumps or the need to eat.

An average 70-kilo (154 lbs.) well-nourished man carries 161,000 kcal of stored energy. Put in perspective, an average well-nourished man has enough stored energy to last more than a month without food.[45] The few hours of energy supplied by a meal pales in comparison. How much more energy would you have locked away in your body if you're more than the average weight?

Sugars are always burned off first before fats. It's the reason why fat burning stops when you eat, there's sugar to be burned. Some experts even argue sugar is toxic, it's why your body gets rid of it. Anyway, I digress. Unfortunately, sugar is less energy dense than fats. A gram of fat has 9 calories, while a gram of carbohydrate, like glucose, has 4 calories.[46] Less than half of fats. In addition, you don't tap on fats until your glycogen stores are depleted. Glycogen stores typically lasts 8-22 hours depending on the person and the person's activities.[47] Until then, you rely on sugar to fuel your body.

Physical activity also depletes glycogen stores. The combination of not consuming anything during the day and physical activity will deplete glycogen stores and cause the body to shift to using fats for fuel. This gives you a stable and more abundant energy source. Burning body fats is simply a more reliable energy source than constantly eating.

"What is that?" I sniffed. My stomach groveled. It's like I smell everything, especially food. My vision seems more acute, more sensitive to movement. I heard a rustle at the front door. "Who's there?" It appears my hearing is better too. At least better at picking up small sounds sneaking behind me. "Monsieur Pong, C'est moi. I didn't know you've arrived." It's the cleaning lady. "Bonjour madame! Do you smell that?" It smells like meat and some breaded carbohydrate with chili, deep fried in vegetable oil. "Smell what monsieur?" The lady asked. I suddenly realized below my flat, two houses away, lunch is being cooked. Up here in my apartment, I may be the only one smelling it.

Evolutionary considerations suggest our bodies are optimized to perform at a food deprived state. Eating three meals a day plus snack is abnormal compared to the eating habits of our ancestors before the Agricultural Revolution. Competition for limited food drove evolution. Individuals with high physical performance in a food-deprived state got food and survived to pass on their genes to the next generation, us.

Generally, exercise and food deprivation activate the cells' adaptive stress response pathways and pathways which enhance organ plasticity and functionality. It also improves cardiovascular stress adaptation and increases the number of synapses in the brain. Think about it. Animals who haven't eaten in weeks need to find food before severe symptoms of starvation sets in. Obviously, it's important for their brain and body to function well in a food-deprived state. Otherwise, they won't find food or have the ability to compete for food with other animals.

Not only are they able to function well but experiments on lab animals showed they perform better in a food-deprived state. Cognitive function, learning, memory, and alertness increased. Mice maintained in an alternate-day fast during a month of treadmill training have better endurance.[48]

In lab animals, food deprivation and exercise stimulated Brain-Derived Neurotrophic Factor (BDNF) in the nerve cells. This protein plays an important role in learning, memory, and the generation of new nerve cells in the hippocampus. BDNF also makes neurons more resistant to stress.[49] When you're food-deprived your neurons (and your entire body) is in a "self-conservation mode." When you eat, your body then shifts to "growth mode." When you're full there's no reason to fight to have food. Heightened senses are not needed anymore because you just ate.

Live a Long Healthier Life

It has been mentioned all over this book, eating one meal a day decreases your risk of contracting chronic diseases. Though I think it's worth briefly mentioning once more.

You may scoff at the mention of diseases like obesity and diabetes because they're mentioned way too often, it seems like everybody gets it and is normal. But it's not. Those diseases don't appear by default. Those diseases are preventable. If you could cut down on consuming too much food, too soon, and too often, your risk goes down. When your risk goes down, you have a shot at living a longer healthier life.

OMAD reduces your relative calorie intake. Calorie restriction has been shown to increase lifespans across the animal kingdom. If you reduce an organism's caloric intake they live longer. It has been tried on yeast, worms, rodents, spiders, insects, rabbits, dogs, and monkeys. Caloric restriction is the only known way (at the time of this writing) of deliberately extending the lifespan of any organism at will.[50] This includes humans.

Members of the Calorie Restriction Society have imposed on themselves a 30% reduced daily caloric intake compared to normal people. After an average of

15 years of reduced caloric intake findings show calorie restriction in humans has the same effect described in long-lived calorie-restricted animals and insects. In addition, calorie restriction, with optimal intake of nutrients decreased metabolic and hormonal risk factors for type 2 diabetes, cardiovascular disease, stroke, cancer, and vascular dementia.[51]

You don't have to count calories. It's too complicated. I know, I used to do it. My aim is to simplify. I don't focus on calorie count because my hunch is it's the effect of food deprivation itself which gives these people and animals their longevity. The orderly breakdown of molecules for energy extends their lifespan. On OMAD, we "deprive" ourselves of food so the body could use its glycogen stores and breakdown fats during the day. A lot of metabolic changes happen when the body shifts from using energy from consuming food constantly to breaking down its food stores for energy. Without food, cells in our body become self-regulating.

In addition, you're consuming fewer calories on OMAD anyway! Not intentionally most of the time. So, no need to count calories for calorie restriction's sake. It's hard to over eat with one meal, the digestive system has physical limits, you know. The simpler you can make your routine the more likely you'll stick to it. I simply eat and eat more if I want, then stop when I'm full–my body tells me when to stop. It's simpler than counting calories.

Help The Environment

"Those corporations are evil! Not only are they feeding us unhealthy food full of toxins, the meat industry destroys and pollutes the environment for profit. Eating meat is needless consumption, it's bad." I've had this conversation about one hundred fifty-two million times already! I looked at this girl I just met as she rolled her organic cigarette with some special paper. She lit it, then took a puff or two. I coughed. "This is why being vegetarian is good. You help the environment and it's healthy. You don't consume all those toxins in meat." I swear, I want to strangle anyone who alleges vague unspecified toxins in food. Just what exactly are these toxins? I thought. She's ideologically driven, moralizes eating, and she mistakenly puts the blame where it doesn't belong. As I coughed and looked at her smoke while she talked about what is healthy, needless consumption, and how humans are destroying the planet, I could only think to myself, she has no clue what she's talking about.

Bear with me as I explain how OMAD helps the planet.

The problem is not food corporations or "the industry." The problem is human consumption. We simply consume way too much. Corporations and "the industry" are simply supplying our demands. If you reduce consumption you help the environment. When we collectively reduce demands for certain products, we reduce the production of those products. Including food. Reduced production means less strain on the environment. Corporations are at the whim of we the consumers, not the other way around. Mass production is simply meeting mass demand. No company on earth would produce something nobody wants to buy. If they do, they go bankrupt.

Being a vegetarian doesn't help reduce consumption because vegetarians need to consume more plants to meet their caloric requirements compared to those who eat meat.

As long as the serving sizes weigh the same, meat has more calories than any plant-based food. A 3oz. (88ml.) serving of lean meat has 180 calories, while a 3oz. serving of lettuce only has 13 calories. Put in perspective, a vegetarian need to consume about 40oz. (1.13 kg) of lettuce to match the calories found in a mere 3oz. of lean meat—and that is lean meat. How much more calories would a serving of fatty meat contain compared to a serving of lettuce?

Consuming more plants to meet your nutritional needs doesn't sound like helping the environment or reducing consumption. Remember consumption drives production. More production means more stress on the environment.

What most people don't know, agriculture is the biggest environmental threat. It has the largest environmental impact than any other human activity. Agriculture uses 50% of the habitable areas of the planet and wastes 60% of the water it uses.[52] Farming is driving the sixth mass extinction of life on Earth[53] whether organic or conventional.

Vegans, vegetarians, and organic-food crazies alike mistakenly blame livestock production for the destruction of the environment, not knowing we're clearing away forests to make way for single crops we prefer eating.

Take the humble avocado. Popularized and hailed in social media and by vegetarians as a superfood, avocados created a huge demand. In the US in 2018, 2.4 million tonnes of avocados were consumed.[54] In 2017 in the UK, demand for avocado rose by 27%.

How can a farmer resist this golden opportunity? The Mexican state of Michoacàn alone produces an estimated $109 million worth of avocados per year. The demand is causing deforestation in Mexico and for rivers in Chile to be diverted to avocado plantations.[55] [56]

Vegetarians could argue all day the meat industry grows grains just for fodder but I would circle back. The industry only grows fodder to increase production to meet the demand of those who eat three meals a day plus snacks.

The problem is not the corporations or "the industry" per se but people's consumption habits. More consumption, more production, equals more impact on the environment. If you want to help the planet, eat one meal a day. Less consumption, equals less impact on the environment.

The Science of One Meal A Day

The Natural Food Regimen

"We'll follow the river up the mountain." My father and his friend took me and my brother out hiking. "If you want to go there…" my father continued pointing to a direction away from the small river. "…remember to leave signs on the trees so you don't get lost." The forest around the river looked nothing like the Eden I was promised as a boy. There were no trees brimming with edible fruits I could recognize. Whatever looked edible produced a sticky sap or hung on high tenuous branches away from reach. Climbing it was out of the question lest you want to be eaten by a blanket of ants before falling to an early grave. There were also no small animals I could easily spear with my stick. Nature is only good on National Geographic, I thought as insects of all sorts bit every inch of my exposed skin.

Whenever I go in nature I notice how little food item there is in the wild, especially those barely touched by humans. Nature is a bitch. It only looks nice in pictures. Just look at the British reality TV show The Island with Bear Grylls—a show where people are forced to live off the land in a remote island in the Pacific. People in the show struggle to find food and cope with the environment. Seeing such shows should make you question the notion of eating three square meals.

Given such environments, ancient people couldn't have eaten the way we do today.

It doesn't make any logical or biological sense to eat three meals a day for survival. We humans came into existence 500,000 - 800,000 years ago[57] but humans only ate at regular intervals roughly 12,000 years ago during the first Agricultural Revolution in 10,000 BC.[58] You should ask yourself, if humans constantly need to eat three meals a day, then how did our primitive ancestors survived? If it were truly necessary to eat three meals, our species would quickly go extinct.

If it were necessary to eat constantly at regular intervals in a 24-hour period, our ancestors' chances of survival would be zero. So it begs the question, how did our species survive in an environment where food is scarce? The answer lies in the ability to not eat for extended periods of time.

Our species evolved from the wild where there's no 24-hour fast food chains, farms, super markets or refrigerators, and where food fights back. Biologically speaking, we haven't changed. We still possess the same stone age body and genetics.

Diseases of Plenty

Civilization brought us plenty of things, one of them is abundance of food. We domesticated plants and animals to suit human preferences. Foods we consider "natural" or "organic" and therefore "healthy" are very different from their non-domesticated counterparts.

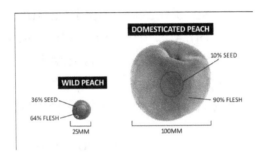

The peach we buy in the market is 4x the size of a wild peach, sweeter, and has more calories. A peach in the wild is 25mm in circumference and has 64% edible flesh. A domesticated peach is 100mm in circumference and has 90% edible flesh. Domesticated corn is 1000x the size of its wild ancestor.[59]

There's also no analogy in nature for food items we eat today. A doughnut (100g) has 452 calories mostly from sugars. An avocado (100g) only has 160 calories. A doughnut beats an avocado, the fruit with the highest calorie count. But this abundance in food and calories have consequences...

Modern diseases or so called diseases of civilization like coronary heart disease, obesity, hypertension, diabetes, epithelial cell cancers, autoimmune disease, and osteoporosis are rare or absent in hunter gatherer societies and other non-westernized civilizations.[60] Those diseases emerged around 12,000 years ago during the first Agricultural Revolution.

The cause of these diseases could be summed up to: too much, too soon, too frequent. The modern human eats too much food than what is needed for survival, eats too soon to consume energy they just ate, and most importantly, they do it too frequently.

Not only do we eat too much, too soon, too often we also don't move as much to acquire food. Our ancestors have to climb tall trees to eat a piece of fruit or spear an auroch to enjoy a piece of steak. In addition, our ancestors cannot store whatever food they could gather and kill. They don't have a fridge. They can only store food [energy] in their fat cells.

The change from hunting and gathering to agriculture was too soon for our ancient stone age bodies to adapt.[61] As a result, we get fat and sick. One meal a day is not the torture people make it out to be. I'd argue it's necessary for us to maintain our health. It's like when Steve Jobs said, "Use it the way it was designed." We evolved in a food-deprived environment. Our stone age bodies are simply not designed for an environment where food is easy to get, plentiful, and contain high calories.

We're not intended to eat three meals a day. When our species started eating constantly we started to suffer from diseases of civilization. From this information and what we know about the effects of food deprivation, we could assume our bodies need to go through cycles of feasting and fasting to be healthy. We need to use our bodies the way it evolved.

Amazing Fats

"It's amazing." I said out loud, half-shocked, as I watched one of the heaviest man on earth. He could barely move on his bed. He reminded me of beached whales. I wonder how many oil lamps he can fuel if you melted his fats down like how Inuits used whale blubber for fuel? I shook the thought and continued watching. It's nicer to watch an English woman talk of the man's diet plan than think of lighting oil lamps with his blubber.

Fats are amazing! It's energy-dense and easy to put on, as most of us know. Our fat cells can expand until it's full and our bodies can create more fat cells to store any excess food energy if need be. We can store an unlimited amount of fats in our body as seen in morbidly obese individuals extricated from their houses with a forklift,[62] as opposed to around 500 grams of sugar in the liver and skeletal muscles.[63] Excess dietary sugars can even be converted to fats in a process called de novo lipogenesis when glycogen stores are full.[64] Our body doesn't throw food energy away.

Even a thin person who has little fat from our perspective is fat compared to other primates. The average primate carries 5-8% body fat, an average thin human hunter-gatherer female has 15-25% body fat, while males would have 10-15% body fat.[65]

This is the reason why OMAD is neither dangerous nor unhealthy. You have fats. You breakdown fats in place of food if you don't eat. Unfortunately, our modern diets don't allow us to breakdown these wonderful fats for energy. We can only use body fats for energy when there's no sugar available for our body to use. We eat too often, too much, and too soon. Not to mention there's way too much simple sugars in an average modern human's diet.

Fats both in and out of my body have been a wonderful thing in my OMAD journey. Externally, I eat it to easily satisfy my caloric requirements. A little goes a long way. Internally, my body burns it for fuel.

Fat Adapted

"Are we there yet?" My little brother asked. We're on a road trip, me, my sister, my brother, and my sister's girlfriend. It's almost nightfall. I was the driver. They all look tired. I know they're on a sugar slump. They ate breakfast, lunch, a snack, a small snack, and another snack a few hours ago. They also took small bites of the food samples in the market. I haven't eaten anything yet. They're cranky and lethargic. I'm still energetic considering I drove all day, ran around, and moved more. "No bro." I answered. "We'll eat as soon as we get to the city. My treat! A little patience. Okay?"

Fat adaptation is the body's ability to use fats as it's main source of fuel. Most people are not fat adapted like our ancestors. People who are fat adapted don't get cranky or lethargic when they have nothing to eat because they can tap into their vast fat reserves. They also don't have energy slumps, their energy is stable throughout the day.

Most people eat diets anchored on carbohydrates. This means instead of burning fats for energy they rely on burning sugars (carbohydrates) for energy. I alluded to this before on our previous chapter. When the supply of sugar dips, energy dips, resulting to lethargy, crankiness, cravings, and inability to focus–experiences most people associate with hunger. To fix this problem and maintain sustained energy levels people eat sugars constantly. They never allow themselves to become fat adapted.

Fats are not bad or undesirable as we imagined it to be. What's bad is when we have too much of it and it affects our health. In our present environment it's not very hard to do. It could easily be remedied if we use fats as fuel instead of accumulating it in our body.

Anyone who does OMAD will eventually become fat adapted.

There's very little reason to believe we're ever going to starve or not have enough energy when we eat only one meal. If the cave man hunted mammoths, fought off sabertooth tigers, and had enough energy to have plenty of sex and babies with one meal a day or less, you'll be fine eating a meal a day with modern high-calorie food.

A Guide To Eating One Meal A Day

How To Eat One Meal A Day

Before you skip meals be sure to read this part of the book *carefully*. There's a method to this. We don't want severe caloric deficits and macronutrient deficiencies. For some of you, I understand the pressing need to lose weight, now! But I'd rather have those who read this book choose their long-term health than obsess with weight loss in the short to medium term.

It's important to remember, getting results from OMAD is a long slow process. Being healthy is not a one-time endeavor; it's a lifetime commitment. Avoid the temptation of eating one meal a day just to lose weight. I know a lot of people want to lose weight badly but you must reframe your thinking. Instead of "weight" think "health." Your goal is more than the number on the scale. If you shift your thinking, your weight will follow your thinking. People are fat because of what they do. What they do is the result of how they think.

Once you decide to go OMAD, you're going to eat one meal a day for the rest of your life. One meal a day will be your standard operating procedure.

I would reiterate, especially if you have medical conditions: I'm not your doctor or a medical professional. Don't do anything crazy. Consult your doctor because you're responsible if something happens to you.

Now, prepare to be amazed at how little your body needs to function well!

There are six steps and four strategies I used to transition from eating multiple meals to eating one meal a day. The steps are:

1. Remove snacks.

2. Eat no carbs for breakfast.

3. Remove breakfast.

4. Replace lunch with a snack-sized meal.

5. Remove lunch.

6. Eat one meal a day.

The strategies we'll use to implement those six steps are:

1. Replace

2. Reduce

3. Remove

4. Eat fats and proteins

We'll first discuss each step and strategy in detail in the succeeding chapters, then we'll summarize so you remember the important points. If you notice, the steps lead to dinner as the sole meal in a 24-hour period. Why dinner will be explained later. These steps are not clear-cut rules; they serve more as guidelines for you to follow. Again, be sensible with this endeavor. Do it gradually. I can't stress it enough, do it gradually. If you don't feel good don't do it. Revert to your regular diet, figure out what went wrong then start again.

The steps assume you eat three major meals and snacks in between. You may have a different idea how to do this based on your diet, habits, and lifestyle. As they say, there's no one way to skin a cat. But I think the steps and strategies would be similar no matter how you go about it.

My Transition To One Meal A Day

We need context before we begin. So let me describe my eating habits before I started OMAD. Let's start when I first took health and fitness seriously.

I was bodybuilding. My diet would be generally described as "clean eating." I cooked my own meals and I bought the best ingredients available to me. Each meal is roughly composed of 45% proteins, 35% carbohydrates, and 20% fats. I ate vegetables and fruits. Lean meats were the foundation of my diet. In addition, I took several supplements I needed for bodybuilding. I ate 6-8 meals per day and consumed around 7,000 calories. I used to get cranky when I delay a meal. I was hungry all the time back then. It was impossible to function with less, or so I thought.

I knew if I wanted to go OMAD, I would have to transition slowly. I suggest you do it slowly too. Nothing drastic. If it takes more than a year or two, so be it. We're doing it for health and longevity. We're not competing with anyone else. We're in it for the long run. We'll be doing this for the rest of our lives.

My transition to one meal a day took about a year or so. You can do it with more time or less time. It doesn't matter, as long as you set the goal of eating one meal a day.

OMAD Nutrition Basics

If you're going OMAD, it's crucial you eat nutrient-dense foods. So it's important to have a rudimentary understanding of nutrition so you know what to eat, reduce, and remove. You'd be surprised how a lot of people diet but have no clue about nutrition. They end up following diet prescriptions and don't know why and how it works or if it even makes any sense!

We need to discuss the basics of nutrition because the basics always apply. The quickest way to gain knowledge about nutrition is understanding macronutrients. There are only three: proteins, fats, and carbohydrates. These are the big words you hear most when people talk about nutrition.

Macronutrients are chemical compounds in food used by your body for energy and bodily functions. You need macronutrients in large quantities, unlike micronutrients which you need in small quantities. Micronutrients (vitamins and minerals) are substances required in trace amounts for normal bodily functions. In food, micronutrients naturally come with macronutrients.

Don't worry too much about micronutrients you need them in very low quantities. It's the macronutrients you need to get right as you need them in large quantities.

One of your OMAD tasks is to examine your meals and categorize each food item into macronutrient categories. Every food item is rich in a specific macronutrient. For example, meats would be mostly protein. Pasta would be carbohydrates. Olive oil would be fats. Categorizing food items like this makes it easier to implement our 3 Rs: replace, reduce, remove.

Proteins

Proteins are large molecules which perform a critical role in your body. They do most of the work in cells and are required for the structure, function, and regulation of tissues and organs.[66] Proteins make up virtually every part of your body from your hair to your heart.

Proteins are made up of smaller organic compounds called amino acids. Your body combines amino acids from food to form proteins. There are three types of amino acids: Essential, nonessential, and conditionally essential amino acids.

Essential Amino Acids - your body can't produce it. It needs to be acquired through food.

Nonessential Amino Acids - your body can produce it even if you don't acquire it through food.

Conditionally Essential Amino Acids - become essential in times of adversity, like in times of illness or stress.

Your body needs 20 amino acids to function properly and form proteins. Of the 20 amino acids, 9 are essential and must be acquired through food on a regular basis.

There are plant sources of proteins but the best source of proteins come from animal products such as meats, seafood, milk, egg whites, and cheese.

You can find small quantities of proteins in plants but I would not recommend depending on plants for your protein intake especially on OMAD, despite what vegetarians and vegans would say. I used to be a vegetarian and did my undergrad thesis on vegetarianism. It's why I can't recommend relying on plants for your protein requirements, unless you want to be bone thin and weak.

To give you an idea, 100 grams of meat has 26 grams of protein. 100 grams of broccoli has 2.8 grams. To get the same amount of protein from broccoli you would have to eat ten times more broccoli. You can't afford to just fill up with broccoli when you're eating one meal a day because you need to eat other food items to take care of both your macronutrient and micronutrient needs.

Most plant proteins are incomplete proteins, they're missing at least one essential amino acid. In addition, plant proteins are not as bioavailable as meat proteins. Plant proteins take longer for your body to use because plant proteins are wrapped in fiber.

Fats

Fats are substances which give the body energy. It's crucial for normal body function. It allows the body to use fat-soluble vitamins,[67] keeps hair and skin healthy, protects organs, and insulates the body.[68] Steroid hormones like testosterone and estrogen are derived from fats. Fats, as mentioned earlier in this book, is also needed for a healthy brain. Again, there's no healthy brain without fats. Fats are essential for life.

Dietary sources of fats are animal fats found in meats and seafood, egg yolk, dairy products, nuts, and plant oils.

Dietary fats could be classified into:

1. Saturated fats

2. Monounsaturated fats

3. Polyunsaturated fats

4. Trans fats

Don't be afraid of fats or go out of your way to avoid it. The only type of fat you should avoid like how you'd avoid lepers are trans fats.

Trans fats are processed fats. Although there are some natural sources of trans fats, most trans fats are formed in an industrial process of adding hydrogen to vegetable oil so it can have a longer shelf life.[69] Thus the name "hydrogenated vegetable oil." I bet you've seen it before on food labels and didn't know what it was.

Trans fats are the worst thing you can eat. It lowers your HDL cholesterol (the "good" fats) and it increases your LDL cholesterol (the "bad" fats). Some dietary sources of trans fats are margarine, vegetable oil, creamer, baked goods, packaged snacks, and some deep fried foods.

In 18 June 2018 the US Food and Drugs Administration banned the use of trans fats on food. They deemed it not generally recognized as safe for human consumption.[70] So it's important you eliminate this kind of fat from your diet.

Carbohydrates

Carbohydrates or saccharides are sugars or starches. They serve as fuel for most organisms.[71] It fuels the central nervous system and energy for working muscles.[72] Unlike fats and proteins, carbohydrates is not needed for any biochemical reactions in the body and you don't need it to survive; its sole purpose is fuel for the body.

Dietary sources of carbohydrates or carbs for short include sugars, fruits, grains, pastries, honey, syrup, and starchy vegetables.

Carbohydrates can be divided into simple and complex carbs. Complex carbs are carbs wrapped in fiber, like those found in fruits and whole grains. Simple carbs are carbs taken out of their fiber wrapping.

When carbs are incased in fiber your body has to breakdown the fiber first before it can get the carbs. This prevents sudden insulin spike and prevents your body from rapidly absorbing sugars. Without the protective fiber, sugars are absorbed at a rapid rate. It causes a sharp rise in insulin level. Frequent rise in insulin level can lead to insulin resistance.

Simple carbs can be found in white rice, pasta, flour, bread, and most processed foods. The simple rule of thumb is: once you take carbs out of its protective fiber it becomes simple.

Note, carbs are not "bad" as online "fitness experts" would like you to believe. You can still eat carbohydrates to quickly replenish glycogen stores, especially after workouts. Eating carbs after workouts help in the post-workout recovery process.

Calories

Calories are not nutrients. I dated a girl once. She was drinking Coke in can. She said, "You know Pong, Coke is also nutritious it has plenty of calories. Look, 150!" My eyes widened as she pointed to the big letters on top of Coke's nutrition facts saying, "150 Calories" in bold letters. I wanted to give her a backhand slap. "They would not put calories prominently if it's not good for you." She continued. In short, she became ineligible for another date.

A calorie is a measure of energy found in food.[73] The three macronutrients contain energy measured in calories. We measure food energy in terms of calories, like how we measure length in centimeters. 1 calorie is equal to heat energy needed to raise the temperature of 1g of water by 1°C.

I wanted to add calories in our discussion of macronutrient since there are people out there who may not know what calories are. Calories, I would repeat, is not nutrition in food but a measure of food energy.

REPLACE

Replace is the first strategy we'll use. Some will find OMAD torture. So before we remove anything from your diet we're going to implement a replacement strategy. To be more specific, we'll be looking at the meal we want to remove and replace carbs with fats and proteins. This will help your body adapt to removing this meal.

Reduce

Reduce is the second strategy in our arsenal. Very few people can skip a meal without feeling awful. Reducing food quantities will help your body acclimatize to skipping regular meals. We want to make the transition from eating three meals a day plus snack to one meal a day as smoothly as possible.

Start by reducing food item quantities until you can comfortably remove it. This results in an overall reduction in meal size. Keep reducing food quantities until you can comfortably remove the entire meal. For example, you can reduce carbs in each meal by 25%. Once your body adapts, reduce it again by 25%. Eat like this until your body adapts to the reduction. You can keep on reducing gradually until you can comfortably remove the meal.

You can use reduction and replacement in tandem. Put more fats and proteins in place of the carbs you just reduced until you have no carbs in the meal. Then you can start reducing proteins and fats. Keep reducing until you can eliminate the entire meal.

Remove

Remove once the quantities are small enough and your body has adapted to a reduced food intake. We can remove either the food item in question or the entire meal. Always remove carbs first. Remove fats and proteins last. You know when you've adapted to a reduced food intake when you can easily not eat the meal you want to remove. If you're not hungry come mealtime you can safely remove said meal.

Eat fats and proteins

Fats and proteins keep you full longer. Eating fats and proteins is one of the best strategies to apply when adapting to OMAD. Fats and proteins don't stimulate insulin production as much as carbs. If you remember, eating carbs stimulate insulin production. Insulin antagonizes hormone-sensitive lipase preventing you from becoming fat adapted.

Eating One Meal A Day Step By Step

In summary the steps to transition from three meals a day to one meal a day are:

1. Remove snacks.

2. Eat no carbs for breakfast.

3. Remove breakfast.

4. Replace lunch with a snack-sized meal

5. Remove lunch.

6. Eat one meal a day.

STEP 1: Remove Snacks

Stop eating snacks. Eat substantial meals rich in proteins and fats, it will keep you full longer, thus eliminating the need for snacks.

To transition from eating multiple meals to eating a single meal, we have to go back to three square meals. This means quitting snacks. Compared to breakfast or lunch snacks are the easiest to quit.

For a lot of people, snack is a carbohydrate-rich easy to eat food item used as a bridge between meals. It's convenient, fast, rewarding, and could be eaten anytime anywhere with minimal effort.

In my opinion, snacks are sources of unnecessary doses of sugar which disrupts fat breakdown. It keeps you stuck in the sugar trap. It's also an easy way to put extra calories which lead to weight gain—I exploited this to get bigger for bodybuilding.

To quit snacks, I ate a decent-sized meal for breakfast and lunch. At first I replaced simple carbs with a smaller quantity of complex carbs (one which has fiber) and ate more fats and proteins. The combination of tough fiber in complex carbs and eating more fats and proteins kept me full longer and helped me stop snacking.

In the morning, I started eating eggs and steel-cut whole oats soaked in water or milk overnight. Eggs with black bread and butter were also an alternative whenever I got tired of eating oats. I skipped honey. For lunch, I ate fatty steaks (either fish or beef) and leafy vegetables drizzled in olive oil and a little bit of black or red rice. Eventually I dropped the oats and rice, I just ate proteins and fats.

Proteins and fats keep you full longer because it's harder to digest. They contain complex molecules which take longer for your body take apart. Meat and fish take as long as two days to fully digest. Complex carbs, like fruits and vegetables high in fiber, take about a day. In contrast, your body can tear through simple carbs, like sugary drinks, candies, and energy bars in a few hours.[74]

STEP 2: Eat No Carbs For Breakfast

Remove carbohydrates from breakfast. Eat proteins and fats instead. Replace carbohydrates with proteins and fats little by little until you've removed all carbohydrates from breakfast.

"It was the last of it and I'm not buying again." I said to myself as I stared at an empty jar of steel-cut oats. It felt odd at the time eating no carbs in the morning. It's like a sin against the breakfast gods. Breakfast, after all, was the most important meal of the day. That was gospel. But I have to escape the sugar trap! It was the first time I'm doing this. "Nobody told me how to do this!" I said out loud as if trying to appease the breakfast gods. I stood in front of my fridge and stared at the food items in it. I had a choice, cheese dipped in olive oil, butter on omelette, or leftover steak from last night. "Steak then." maybe with butter on top, I said.

Some epidemiological research say having breakfast high in rapidly available carbohydrates (simple carbs) increase the risk of metabolic syndrome[75] like obesity and diabetes.

An epidemiological study is not the most robust science, but based on what we know, simple carbs like sugar definitely plays a big factor on our health or lack thereof. Some might argue sugar is not the problem, excess calorie intake is.[76] No matter how you look at it, breakfast can be both a source of simple rapidly absorbing carbs and excess calories.

Take special notice of hidden sugars when removing carbs from your morning meal. Many processed food may seem purely fats and proteins (like bacon and sausage) but may contain sugars upon closer inspection of the ingredient list. Always read food labels, especially the ingredient list.

Aside from the obvious sugar, honey, and syrup, sugars come in many names, from the chemical-sounding "neotame," to the benign-sounding "fruit juice concentrate," to the downright deceptive "organic evaporated cane juice." It also hides in words ending in "-ose," "-ides," or "-ol." Glucose, sucralose, lactose, galactose, monoglycerides, polyglycerides, disaccharides, glucitol, malitol, and xylitol.[77] Those are all sugars.

People like it sweet but they don't want to see the word "sugar" on their food label. So manufacturers remove "sugar" and replaced it with something else sweet. A simple rule of thumb is: if it's sweet it must be sugar, therefore don't eat.

Remember, carbohydrates are not only sugar. Carbohydrates are also starches. Rice, pasta, bread, crackers, and cereals are sugars. All types of carbohydrates are broken down in the body into glucose (sugar). Remember not to eat these for breakfast so you can eventually escape the sugar trap and remove breakfast.

STEP 3: Remove Breakfast

You don't need to eat breakfast. Just quit it. Your body can make you breakfast.

"Do I have to?" I pondered one early morning as I stared in my food morgue, the fridge. Pieces of dead plants and animals in sealed glass containers or ziplock bags lined the shelves. Neatly aligned and organized just like a morgue. It's odd to think of food like this. I wasn't hungry, it made all the difference. I don't know of anyone who woke up hungry. I know people can be thirsty when they wake up but hungry? Yet for some reason I have to spend time and money to buy and consume a morning meal. I thought the idea of stuffing my face with food first thing in the morning when I wasn't even hungry was ridiculous, especially when I have a million things to do. "Do I have to eat breakfast? I think not." The decision was easy.

Removing breakfast made plenty of sense based on what I learned. *"Breakfast is the most important meal of the day"* is one of the biggest health myths people believe. You've been given this advice before, eating breakfast will help you lose weight because it boosts your metabolism and it helps you avoid overeating later. This is not true. In fact, eating breakfast may have the reverse effect.[78] Even at face value, eating more to lose weight sounds stupid. You can't eat more and expect to lose weight. Calories don't magically disappear, you know.

The breakfast myth came from breakfast cereal companies.[79] Studies demonstrating breakfast eaters are healthier than non-breakfast eaters are funded by Kellogg's[80] and Quaker Oats. Quaker not only sponsored one of these famous studies it also contributed to the study design and edited the manuscript.[81] This may not automatically mean the studies are wrong but based on what you now know, I think you should be highly skeptical.

Breakfast should be easy to quit (in theory at least) because your body makes your own breakfast when you wake up, remember the dawn effect? You have this marvelous liver which produces all the sugar you need. Besides, are you ever ravenously hungry when you get out of bed? If you followed the previous steps, you won't have problems removing breakfast from your routine. The previous step is a preparation for this step. I suggest using the time you gained from removing breakfast to do something else.

You must quit coffee too! I used to love coffee. I used to fight tooth and nail for this stuff. But I don't recommend it anymore. The point of eating one meal a day is to consume nothing before the meal at the end of the day. Apply the same strategies: reduce then remove.

I know there are plenty of studies about coffee being healthy and how black coffee doesn't break your fast etc., but coffee has caffeine which have effects on the body. We'll discuss coffee in detail later.

You don't have to quit the coffee habit now. You can quit coffee once you mastered OMAD. Just remember you have to eventually quit it. Coffee withdrawal takes about 3 days. Once you pass 3 days, you won't have coffee cravings anymore.

STEP 4: Replace Lunch With a Snack-sized Meal

Eat a fat and protein-rich snack-sized meal instead of a full meal for lunch. In addition, consume no carbs with this meal.

"Is that creamer?" "No. Butter." I replied as I mixed a heaping teaspoon of butter in my espresso. "What are you doing buddy? Is this all you're going to eat for lunch?" He pointed at my espresso's saucer of three different cheeses and half a piece of saltine. "Buddy, why don't you eat like a man!" Proudly showing me his plate of rice, beans, and ground meat. My next door neighbor, a good friend of mine, decided to eat lunch with me today. I pointed at his shirtless chest and said, "And have manly boobs like you?" We laughed.

Removing lunch will be different from removing breakfast and snacks because lunch is a more substantial meal. According to various calorie recommendations, a typical lunch would be anywhere from 400-700 calories.[82] [83] [84] [85] No matter which expert you ask, lunch accounts for a large chunk of your caloric intake. Skipping lunch will not be easy. I know it wasn't easy for me. Gradually reducing lunch size over time will get you adapted to skipping lunch.

The same strategies apply here. Before replacing a full lunch with a "snack" ease yourself to eating no lunch by replacement, reduction, and eating fats and proteins. Replace carbs first little by little before reducing lunch to snack size.

Take the same actions you took in the previous steps. Replace carbs with proteins and fats. Gradually reduce food quantity. When your body gets used to the reduce food quantity, reduce it again. Keep reducing and adapting until you're eating so little you can comfortably not eat lunch.

For this step, I used to eat left over meat from dinner and some leafy vegetables or broccoli drizzled in olive oil. I removed my favorite starch, rice, little by little from lunch until I was eating only the proteins and fats. This was also eventually reduced to insignificant quantities. When I got used to it, I got rid of it too. I started buttering my coffee and eating cheese with a saltine. As my body adapted, I cut the saltine in half, then a fourth. I ended up having a buttered espresso and cheese for lunch. I kept reducing the amount of cheese until I only had a shot of buttered espresso. At this stage, I reduced coffee intake in the same manner. You may want to do it differently, but I think you get the main idea. Replace, reduce, eliminate, and eat fats and proteins.

In addition to lunch being one of the most substantial meal people eat, lunch is also associated with social calls. It's difficult for most people to say no, especially when everybody around them is eating lunch. In a professional environment, a lot of things are talked about over lunch. Alliances are forged, deals are made, etc.

By eating a smaller meal at lunchtime, you not only help your body adapt to eating one meal a day. You also help the people around you adjust to your new eating habit. Surely, they will ask you why you're eating the way you do. It's the perfect time for you to explain the benefits of OMAD and tell them to read my book! You'll be the focal point of the conversation. By discussing how you skip meals and how you'll eat one meal a day in the future, you turn yourself into an expert instead of a lunchtime outcast.

STEP 5: Remove Lunch

You don't need lunch. You have enough energy stored in your body to last you more than a month. Skipping lunch will not make a dent on those energy stores.

"Gone." I said. I was thinking of last month's last slice of Camembert, my favorite cheese, as I gulp my buttered half espresso. I could not remember when I last ate lunch like a man, as my friend would put it. "There's not even any sense to this espresso anymore." I've been talking to myself a lot at lunchtime. I wasn't hungry and I felt, uh, normal for the rest of the day. I think it's time to quit lunch or whatever this is.

I chose to live close to work. The office and my flat was separated by a 5-minute walk and ten flights of stairs, one way. At lunchtime while everybody stuffed themselves with food, I went home to edit podcasts or prepare show notes for the week's podcast episode. If I'm not taking care of podcasting, I was doing research about anything related to health. Whatever mountain of task needs to be done for my side projects, I do some of it in the hour I gained not eating lunch. When I tell people I work a full-time job, freelance, do podcasts, make YouTube videos, read books, and exercise four to five times a week they often think what I do is impossible or I'm lying. I was always tempted to say, it's impossible for you because you eat all the time.

Consuming no carbs in the previous step is crucial. We want the body to be fat adapted before removing lunch. Once you quit lunch you'll be relying solely on your body's energy stores. It's important you're fat adapted before you quit lunch.

In the previous step you ate a "snack" or a small fat and protein-rich meal, then reduced it little by little. At this point you should be eating so little for lunch you could just as easily eat nothing. If you're eating very little for lunch for some time now you won't even feel hungry come midday. So just skip lunch. If not, go back to the previous steps.

Before you quit lunch, make sure you're comfortable with eating just a small amount of food at lunchtime. Your midday food intake should be almost nothing before you quit lunch, like my half shot of buttered espresso. Don't rush yourself. How you adapt to food reduction is different from another person so take as much time as you need. Go back to the previous steps if you must.

Once you quit lunch, you're officially on OMAD.

STEP 6: Eat One Meal A Day

Once you start eating one meal a day, you'll be eating like this for the rest of your life. When we say "one meal a day" we mean consuming nothing (other than water) before this meal.

CONGRATULATIONS, You're eating one meal a day!

You'll have some challenges in the beginning, physiological, psychological, and social. I find the hardest part of OMAD is the social aspect. Since everybody eats all the time you'll face constant challenges. People will always try to tempt you to eat. They will offer you food. They'll even offer free lunch just to spite you or test your resolve. They'll ask you a lot of questions. They will tell you all the reasons why you're wrong. But stand firm. This book has given you the knowledge and the reasons why eating one meal a day is more sensible than eating three or more meals a day. Use meal times to talk about it, instead of giving in to what everybody says. If you want extraordinary health you can't do the ordinary things ordinary people do.

People will discourage you from OMAD not because they're a-holes but because they feel uncomfortable knowing they may be doing something wrong. Unlike you, they never questioned their meals or their habits. Worst, by explaining what you learned in this book they might've realized their eating habits might've caused them some health issues or they might've believed lies or practiced bad nutrition science. It may be too late for them, they fear. Be patient with these people. It's not OMAD or you, it's them.

You can eat as much as you want and eat whatever you want. Eat until you're full then stop. Go for several servings if you want. Eat until you can't. Your body has evolved for millions of years. It knows when you should stop eating.

A lot of people are scared of indigestion or acid reflux when they eat a lot. I think these are caused by people not eating according to how we humans evolved in the wild, this is of course barring people with health issues. As always, be sensible. If you know you have problems don't go eating until you drop just because some guy wrote a book. Go slow, see how your body reacts, then adjust to how your body reacts. Your body knows what it needs if you could only listen and interpret what it's saying.

I let my body dictate how much to eat, then I stop when it says so. I'm also mindful of how my stomach fills up. I intentionally chew my food and put a lot of awareness on the taste, texture, and scent of my food. This way, I don't mindlessly shovel food in my mouth.

Since you're eating one meal per day, it's important to get all the nutrients and consume all the calories you need in this single meal. Eat fruits, vegetables, carbs, proteins, and fats. Eat full course meals. Appetizers, main courses, and desserts. If you want to drink alcohol, I suggest you take it while eating or after the appetizer. It's not wise to drink alcohol on an empty stomach. Enjoyment of food is part of being healthy.

In addition to not eating trans fats and reducing simple carbs, quit processed foods. In the loose sense of the word, a lot of the food items we eat are "processed." Olive oil, for example, is processed from olives. Cooking is a process. What we're referring to are food items which went through a series of mechanical and/or chemical processes to change or preserve it. If it comes packaged, it must be processed. It's best to avoid even if you can eat whatever you want on OMAD. A lot of these food items have little in terms of nutrition. When you eat only one meal nutrient density is important. Otherwise you'll feel cravings and hunger. It means you're missing some nutrients.

OMAD Steps Summary

Here is a quick summary of the steps you need to take to transition from multiple meals to one meal a day. Bookmark this page for easy reference.

Step 1: Remove snacks

Stop eating snacks, especially carbohydrate-rich snacks. It only makes you hungry and prevents your body from breaking down fats for energy. Eat a decent-sized protein and fat rich meal. It will keep you full longer and remove the need for snacks.

Step 2: Eat no carbs for breakfast

Eat fats and proteins for breakfast. Eliminate all carbs gradually. Carbs only make you reach for a snack mid-morning. Carbohydrates in the morning break the prior night's fasting period while you were asleep. Fasting is when your body is breaking down its energy stores to fuel itself. It's a time when fats are broken down. Take advantage of this golden opportunity to teach your body to be fat adapted.

Step 3: Remove breakfast

Stop eating breakfast. Your body can make your own breakfast. If you can't eliminate breakfast, ease yourself by implementing our strategies. Gradually reduce the amount of food until you're eating next to nothing. Then quit breakfast once it's small enough to be removed.

Step 4: Replace lunch with a snack-sized meal

Eat a snack-sized fat-rich and protein-rich meal for lunch. This step will help you eventually quit lunch. Eating more proteins and fats and little to no carbs help you become fat adapted. Like in the previous steps, if you can't yet replace a full meal with a snack-sized meal, replace and reduce, then remove.

Step 5: Remove lunch

Stop eating lunch. You don't need lunch. Your body has enough energy to last you more than a month without food. Skipping lunch will not make a dent on your energy stores. You just need to tap it by not eating. If you can't quit lunch yet, go back to Step 4 and eat fats and proteins. Reduce then remove. Take your time because once you eliminate lunch, you're officially on OMAD.

Step 6: Eat one meal a day.

You're eating one meal a day. We consume nothing but water before this meal. No snack. No coffee. No tea. Definitely no solid food. The only thing we put in our mouths prior to this meal is water. Eat a full course meal. Enjoy your meal. Eat whatever you want in as much quantity as you want. Stop when you're full or when you're done with your meal.

Tips And Tricks

Here are some tips and tricks to help you eat one meal a day.

Drink plenty of water.

Drink around three to four liters of water a day. More if you're active or when it's hot. This is important especially when you're just starting out. Drinking water eases hunger. Some say thirst and hunger can be confused. At times, you may just be thirsty instead of hungry.

Deal with hunger.

Dealing with hunger will be a challenge for most people. Hunger is not permanent. It comes in waves during the day. If you feel hunger, let it pass. Eventually, it goes away on its own. Though, it may come back later in the day. Engaging in an activity will help you forget hunger. Remember, hunger felt close to meal times is learned. You're unlearning hunger if you let it pass.

If it helps, I'll share this litany I borrowed and modified from Frank Herbert's The Litany Against Fear in his Dune novel:

I must not eat.

Hunger is the OMAD-killer.

I will not eat.

I will allow it to pass over me and through me

When it has gone to past,

Only I will remain.

I just close my eyes and repeat this litany until the hunger passes. It helped me go through 3-4 days of fasting, it may help you get through hunger.

If you can let hunger pass, the one meal you'll eat will be wonderful. Hunger is the best sauce, as my Russian friend would always say.

I read a meme once, it said something to the effect of "hunger are fats screaming for mercy as they slowly die." Funny, but do whatever it takes to go OMAD.

Start eating one meal a day when you don't have energy-demanding activities.

It's best to quit eating lunch when you don't have high-energy activities. I started eating one meal a day when I was on vacation—one which involved a lot of sitting on transportation. Use down times to start OMAD or implement one of the steps.

Eat-all-you-can buffets are amazing!

From time to time, especially when people want to eat out, I always suggest to go on an eat all you can buffet. Being on OMAD, I can eat whatever I want and at amazing quantities. You'll get your money's worth in an eat-all-you-can buffet in addition to tasting different foods. People who say I don't enjoy food or life on OMAD don't know what they're missing. Let me see them eat 7-8 plates with bacon, cheese, buttered breads, and 4-5 plates of dessert... this is how I do it and I definitely enjoy it.

Don't eat processed foods.

Avoid processed foods. It's usually a source of trans fats and excess sugars. Processed food items may contain chemical preservatives which are not favorable to health. It would be best to avoid.

Eat food as close to its natural state.

To ensure the nutritional quality of the food you eat, eat foods close to its natural state. Avoid foods which were processed with chemicals, no matter how minimally it was done. Err on the conservative side. If you're not sure don't eat it. There are other food items out there.

Eat more fats.

Fats are your friends. Eat a big meal with fats. If you're losing too much weight or if you need more energy, add more fats to your meals. It can quickly help you meet your caloric requirements. Don't be afraid of fats and fatty meats–fats and proteins are needed to repair your body. These food items will give you plenty of calories.

I like to drizzle olive oil on my food to increase my caloric intake. I also opt for fatty meats, especially beef with a good marbling on it.

Eat a full course meal.

Eat well and enjoy. Eat appetizers. Eat large main courses with salads. Eat desserts. Eating a full course meal will give you variety and help you get different nutrients. The variety also helps you eat more. We tend to quickly reduce hunger and feel full with savory foods but by introducing a course with a different flavor we can eat more.[86] It's crucial to eat more to meet daily caloric requirements and macronutrient needs.

"Front Loading"

When eating a full course meal, eat the most nutrient-dense food and course first. Usually, the main course is the most nutrient dense, followed by appetizer, then dessert. When eating the main course eat proteins and fats first before your complex carbs. Front loading, or putting the most nutrient-dense food up front, ensures you fill yourself up with the nutrition you need. Proteins and fats are more important than carbohydrates, those two have vital functions in the body. Carbs are not essential for any biochemical reactions in the body.

You can eat sweets!

You can eat simple carbs to conclude the meal. You can eat a dessert even when you're full from the first courses you ate. Sugar stimulates the stomach's relaxation reflex. This decreases the pressure inside the stomach and thereby reduces the feeling of being full[87] so you can eat more if you want. The relaxation reflex may also help reduce the feeling of being stuffed.

Eating carbohydrates after exercising or after a whole day of work is also needed to replenish glycogen stores in the skeletal muscles and liver. Eating sweets at the very end of the day also feels like a reward. We need this to psychologically tell ourselves we've done a good job working and not eating during the day. Most people will avoid dessert, but since you're on OMAD indulge. Reward yourself so you reinforce the OMAD behavior. Sweets stimulate the reward centers of your brain.

Eat as much as you want.

We want to consume all the nutrients and calories we need in a single meal. So eat as much as you want. Go for second and third servings. Like warriors on a feast after winning the day, eat until you're full, then stop. You can eat whatever you want and as much as you want but it doesn't mean eating 1-pound bags of M&M and jars of cookies for dinner followed by a can of cola. Be sensible.

Eat a variety of colors and flavors.

Make your plate as colorful as possible. Food's natural color indicates nutrition found in them. Yellow and orange-colored fruits and vegetables contain beta-carotene. Violets and blue-colored fruits and vegetables have polyphenols.

Opt for flavorful dishes. Add herbs and spices on your food when you cook. Like colors, the flavors in food indicate the chemical compounds found in them. The more flavorful [and colorful] the dish is the more chemical compounds it has which may be beneficial to health.

Eat cooked foods and cook your own food.

The process of cooking food makes nutrients more bioavailable. When you cook, you make it easier for the digestive system to absorb the nutrients in food. It also increases the calories you can absorb. When you eat one meal a day, every food item you put in your mouth should count. If you can, cook your own food. When you cook your food you have control over your nutrition. The food you put inside your body is simply too important for you to delegate to somebody else.

Do the groceries on Fridays.

Do your groceries on Friday. There are usually fewer people on Friday compared to weekends. Buying food on Friday also means your food don't have to sit too long in the fridge before you cook it over the weekend.

Cook all your food at one time then store.

After shopping for food on Friday, cook it the following day. I found, cooking food whether it's for the day or for the week takes almost the same time. To economize time batch process, cook for the coming week. Use glass containers to store food in the fridge. Glass is inert and doesn't interact with food. Plastic may release harmful chemicals in your food, not a good idea if you're storing food for the week. In addition, keep your fridge at 4° C (40° F) or lower. This prevents bacterium from growing. Be aware of scent and color change on food. If you're not sure, don't eat.

Cheat from time to time.

If you can get this right 98-99% of the time, it doesn't hurt to sometimes deviate. If you want to eat ice cream, go ahead. Eat the entire pint if you must! Eat cake with it if you want. Eat the junk you want. Then stop. Don't turn it into a cheat day. As long as you don't do it on a regular basis and as long as it's within the context of one meal, go ahead knock yourself out!

You can eat more than one meal from time to time too. Though don't eat more than once with junk in both meals. I recommend eating healthy foods if you must eat more than once.

Our body adapts to what we do. Cheating from time to time is intended to break the pattern and create different stimuli. Alternatively, instead of cheating from time to time, you could do a fast. Skip eating for a day or two. It accomplishes the same thing as cheating but with the benefit of autophagy which we'll discuss later.

Why Dinner?

One argument I usually get is you should not eat anything at night or in the evening. There are plenty of beliefs surrounding this, some of the common ones are:

Belief: *"It's not healthy to eat at night."*

On what basis? None. This is a vague belief bordering superstition. It's like when old people say getting wet by the rain causes colds, as if rain itself causes colds. You can intentionally shower under the rain and not get sick.

Belief: *"If you eat at night, you'll get fat."*

Not true. A calorie eaten at night is processed the same way as a calorie eaten during the day. Your body doesn't magically convert calories into fats just because you ate at night.

Belief: *"You won't have time to fully digest your food before sleep."*

As you know some food items are not fully digested until 2-3 days. Should I wait 2-3 days before I sleep so I could fully digest my food properly?

Argument: *"Your body is less insulin sensitive at night."*

There's evidence to back this claim. However, it doesn't mean your body is not sensitive to insulin at all—we'd be dead if that was true. It's just less sensitive not insensitive. Being in a fasting state for at least 20 hours makes you more sensitive to insulin anyway.

Any action we do requires energy. We know energy from glucose wanes and must be topped frequently. Topping up with glucose requires eating and eating requires time. We also know in the presence of insulin (stimulated by glucose intake), we can't break down fats. Eating at the end of the day allows our bodies to breakdown fats for a steady stable source of energy during the day and by breaking down fats we effectively manage our weight. This is why dinner as the sole meal of the day makes sense. We also maximize time for daily activities when we eat at day's end.

We humans are diurnal creatures, we're active during the day and sleep at night. Gaining back a few hours during the day on OMAD is a slight edge in a competitive world where everybody barely has time for anything. Deferring food related activities allows for uninterrupted work.

I find focus and momentum for work already difficult, no need to make it more difficult with mealtime interruptions. In addition, eating stimulates the parasympathetic nervous system (PSNS). It's the part of the autonomic nervous system responsible for the rest and digest or feed and breed response of the body.[88] The PSNS conserves energy and has a slowing down effect which we don't need during the day.

On the other hand we have the sympathetic nervous system (SNS), it's the antagonist of the PSNS. The SNS is responsible for the fight or flight response. Think of the SNS as the opposite of the PSNS. The sympathetic nervous system is responsible for priming the body for action, particularly in survival situations.[89] By not eating you make sure the PSNS doesn't antagonize SNS activities in the body.

When you work you need to be primed for action. As diurnal creatures it's during the day we need the sympathetic nervous system activity at maximum, why blunt it with a meal just as everybody else? Blunt it by eating at the end of the day to stimulate the parasympathetic nervous system's rest and digest activities, it's when we need it most. I opt to use my body's natural tendencies. Work to bring home the bacon during the day, then relax and enjoy my bacon in the evening–SNS activity during the day, PSNS activity in the evening when I'm about to sleep.

Like ancient warriors, fight when it's time to fight. Relax when it's time to relax. From this perspective, it only makes sense to eat at the end of the day.

What To Eat?

My lover gained weight. Europeans don't eat rice everyday. Rice is a staple in my diet. It reminded me of a diet story I liked... One day two lions were talking on top of a hill overlooking the savannah. "Hey, I heard those elephants live long on their vegetarian diet," said one of the lions. "Yeah, they told me all the benefits of eating only plant foods." Said the other. They talked for a while about the pros and cons of going vegetarian. They concluded it was good. So they decided to eat a vegetarian diet like the elephants. After a few months on the diet, both lions died. I gave my lover's body an examining look. I kinda like it. Her fats are distributed in all the right places. But I ought to change our food for her sake. "Where are you going?" She asked as I suddenly stood up. "I'm going to the market."

There's no one diet for everybody. What works for me may not work for you. We have different activities and fitness levels, thus our nutritional and caloric needs will be different. Our propensity for diseases is also different. Genetic differences play a big factor.

Some do well on a vegetarian diet, some don't do so well on it. Some will do better on a high-fat, high-protein carnivore diet, some won't. I can eat all the rice I want and not gain weight, others become fat after a few weeks.

I will not give food prescriptions here. It's simply impossible for me to design a diet to fit everyone. But maybe, I could tell you what I eat and how I approach eating. You can take it as a starting point and modify it to suit your particular needs.

When it comes to what to eat, you can eat whatever you want at whatever quantity you can. The only hard rule is strictly consume nothing except water before the one meal.

I eat a full course meal. I have a main course, an appetizer, and a dessert. I eat in that particular order. I eat the most nutrient dense course or food item first. This assures I consume as much nutrients as I can before I feel full.

Don't shy away from desserts and carbs. Once out of the sugar trap, I found cravings for something sweet is usually an indicator I need more calories (food energy). So I either eat more food or I simply indulge in a dessert—it's usually very caloric and contains fats and sugar which are pleasurable for us humans to eat.

You don't have to strictly follow this book like gospel. If you're looking a little gaunt, maybe you should add another course or eat something before and after workout sessions. Maybe even eat a hearty breakfast with your family from time to time. It doesn't hurt to break the routine on some occasions, just don't make a habit of it.

When I'm losing too much weight, I eat two appetizers. A small one before the main course and another one after the main course. Sometimes, I eat a banana or two with peanut butter before and after workouts especially if I'm losing weight. Another thing I like doing is mixing butter on hot rice. The combination is not only delicious, it's also very high in calories which would make me gain weight.

If you're gaining weight maybe lay off the sweets and reduce calories. Strictly eat one meal a day and fast for a few days every quarter. Maybe even drop all your carbs entirely! It all depends on what you want to achieve. See what works for you and what doesn't work for you. Do more of what works and don't do what doesn't work. There's no one diet for all as there's no one body alike. Except maybe twins.

So here's how I eat...

Extra Appetizer: Added when I'm losing too much weight. Usually bananas with peanut butter or any nut butter. Fistfuls of nuts would also do. I also like eating pita bread with humus. Crackers and cheese or any pâté are also good. Salad drizzled with a simple vinaigrette would also be an option here. From time to time I eat a good shawarma or a small pizza as an appetizer.

Main Course: Meats, complex carbs, at least 3 different types of vegetables, drizzled with olive oil or sometimes I butter my carbs. Sometimes I go for two or three servings, especially when I did a lot of physical activities during the day. I just eyeball the ratios but typically my plate looks like this:

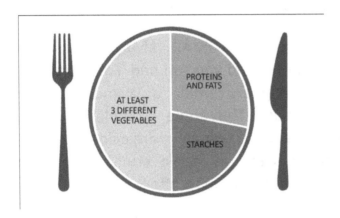

Appetizer: Pita bread with humus, butter, or cheese. If not pita, I eat nuts or whatever appetizer I want to eat. Sometimes I like eating a good salty cheese on a buttered freshly baked bread for appetizer. I like eating bread and salted butter when I'm losing too much weight.

Dessert: If a slice of cake or a cookie is available, I'd have it as dessert. On rare occasions I crave, so I go out of my way to eat ice cream or rice cakes until I'm sick of it. I normally won't have those cravings again for a long time after a binge. Most of the time I just eat fruits or a spoon or three of peanut butter or any nut butter.

Sometimes I skip the dessert when my love handles start to get a bit fatty.

I like sweets. It tastes good and it quickly replenishes glycogen stores after workout sessions or after a day of physical activities. It aids in post-workout recovery, this is why I eat a dessert or carbs in general.

When it comes to OMAD, always choose the most nutrient dense food you can find. For example, I would choose an apple crumble a la mode instead of a chocolate cake. The apple crumble a la mode has apples, spices, and contain more calories. Compared to a chocolate cake, an apple crumble a la mode for dessert has much more to offer.

Another example would be, if I have a choice between a lean steak or a marbled steak, I'd go for the marbled steak. It contains more fats which means more calories. If I have a choice between jasmine rice vs black rice, I'd choose black rice. Lettuce vs spinach, I choose spinach. It's all about choosing foods with more nutrition. Remember, color and flavor equals chemical compounds which may be beneficial for health.

It's very important to note, I'm physically active. I barely sit. I work on a standing desk. I walk as much as I can instead of using vehicles. In the Philippines, I used to live 20-30 minutes walk (one way) from the grocery store. I walk to the grocery then walk back with food for the week in my backpack and grocery bags. I use the stairs more than elevators and escalators. In addition, I workout 3-4 times a week. Sometimes 5-6. I tend to lose weight because of these activities. I'm also muscular. Muscles are bioactive, they burn energy just by being there. More muscles more energy needed to maintain those muscles.

Your food choices will depend on your particular needs. As I've said before, this is not gospel. Be sensible. If you're looking a bit gaunt break OMAD and eat more. If you're gaining weight go back to OMAD, exercise, and fast. You don't have to follow OMAD just because. Remember our body adapts to what we do.

To be of better use to you, here's a list of the range of food items I usually buy. In writing this book, I noticed I usually buy the same items over and over. This list is not in any particular order. Nutrition facts are per 100g of the food item, unless stated otherwise.

PROTEINS AND FATS

ITEM	PROTEIN	FATS	CARBS	CALS.
Eggs (large)*	6g	5g	0.6g	78
Beef	25g	19g	0g	271
Pork	23g	4.5g	0g	130
Chicken	31g	3.6g	0g	165
Milk Fish	21g	6.7g	0g	148
Salmon	20g	13g	0g	208
Tuna Can (water)	24g	3g	0g	128
Bacon	37g	42g	1.4g	541
Butter	0.9g	81g	0.1g	717
Cream	2.7g	19g	3.7g	196
Tofu	8g	4.8g	1.9g	76
Olive Oil**	0g	14g	0g	119
Avocado Oil**	0g	14g	0g	124
Almonds	21.26g	50.65g	19.74g	578
Cashews	18.22g	43.85g	31.19g	553
Wall Nuts	15.23g	65.21g	13.71g	654
Peanuts	28.03g	52.5g	15.26g	599

VEGETABLES

ITEM	PROTEIN	FATS	CARBS	CALS.
Broccoli	2.8g	0.4g	7g	34
Avocado	2g	15g	9g	160
Spinach	2.9g	0.4g	3.6g	23
Pumpkin	1g	0.1g	7g	26
Cauliflower	1.9g	0.3g	6g	25
Cabbage	1.3g	0.1g	6g	25
Carrots	0.9g	0.2g	10g	41
Chayote	0.8g	0.1g	4.5g	19
Green Beans	1.8g	0g	7g	31
Snow Peas	2.8g	0g	7.5g	42
Sprouted Beans	6g	0.7g	13g	67
Mung Beans	24g	1.2g	63g	347
Green Beans	1.8g	0.1g	7g	31
Chick Peas	19g	6g	61g	364
Lentils	9g	0.4g	20g	116
Bitter Melon	3.6g	0.2g	7g	34
Eggplant	1g	0.2g	6g	25
Kale	4.3g	0.9g	9g	49

167

FRUITS & SWEETS				
ITEM	PROTEIN	FATS	CARBS	CALS.
Banana (Med)*	1.3g	0.4g	27g	105
Dragon Fruit	1.2g	0g	13g	60
Mango	0.8g	0.4g	15g	60
Papaya	0.6g	0.1g	9.8g	39
Pineapple	0.5g	0.1g	13g	50
Peanut Butter**	8g	15g	6g	188
Almond Butter**	6.8g	18g	6g	196
*Approx. 7"	2 tbsp				

STARCHES				
ITEM	PROTEIN	FATS	CARBS	CALS.
Black Rice*	6g	0g	48g	213
Red Rice*	4g	0g	48g	200
Red Beets	1.6g	0.2g	10g	43
Potatoes	2g	0.1g	17g	77
Sweet Potatoes	1.6g	0.1g	20g	86
Purple Yams	1g	0.1g	27g	140
Plantains	1.3g	0.4g	32g	122
*1cup (220g) Cooked				

OTHERS

- Various herbs and spices

- Dried mushroom for flavor

- Sea salt

- Soy Sauce

- Vinegars

Various recipes can be created with these food items, but I'm lazy. I prefer not to spend too much time in the kitchen though I like cooking. Like with eating, you can cook whatever you want and however you want. You can do whatever recipe you want to do. Season with whatever you see fit but choose your food well. No processed foods and no trans fats. Be sensible with adding salt, when in doubt err on less salt.

My primary purpose for cooking is to make food more digestible and to kill pathogens. You can make it as fancy as you want or as simple as you want. I prefer simple. I didn't go OMAD only to spend inordinate amounts of time in the kitchen concocting some vaguely special meal. If I want something really special, I eat out. I love those eat all you can buffets. I can eat as much as I want for a decent price.

I usually eat about 0.5-1 kg (1.1-2.2 lbs) of meat a week–different types of animal meats, including seafood. In terms of cooking, I season my proteins with a bit of salt, pepper, and the appropriate spices. I heat my pan, put oil on it. Drop the seasoned protein in. Cook. Turn. Cook. Add dried herbs of choice. Done.

When I feel motivated, I chop onions and garlic. I cut the protein in small pieces then sauté the meat with onions and garlic. Add a bit of herbs and spices. Done.

The less time you expose plant foods to heat the more you preserve their nutrition. I typically drop vegetables in boiling water for 3 minutes. Let cool or dunk in cold water. Done. This is a habit I developed living in Haiti to avoid rampant food-borne illnesses. Boiling water kills pathogens. I'm one of those rare individuals who lived in Haiti and left without parasites.

My staple is black or red rice. I just boil it. Nothing fancy. Same goes for other starches like sweet potatoes and purple yams. Just boil and drizzle with olive oil when you're ready to eat. Sometimes I slather my carbs with butter.

I add cinnamon to my rice. I like the taste and there are some studies which suggest cinnamon helps you control your blood sugar—I don't know for sure, but it doesn't hurt to add flavor on an otherwise bland starch.

I store my food in sealed glass containers in my food morgue, the fridge. Glass doesn't interact with food and has none of the hormone-disputing chemicals which leach into food like with plastic containers. The tight lid minimizes exposure to air, thus limiting oxidation of nutrients. Keeping the fridge in the proper temperature slows down the degradation of nutrients and stops bacterial growth. Food usually stays good for five days. This method has worked for me for years. Give it a try.

Although nutrients in food degrade with time, I don't worry too much about it. My prime concern is meeting my caloric and macronutrient needs. Macronutrients don't degrade like micronutrients and other compounds. It's the reason why you can cook and eat rice sitting in the shelves for months and still get carbs. It's the reason why beef jerky still has proteins despite time passing it by. It's the reason why aged cheese still contains fats despite the aging process. If you're concerned with micronutrients you can take a multivitamin pill.

A Special Note on Coffee

My hands were shaking as I wiped the sweat from my upper lip. "Buddy, another one?" My friend asked. "Sure! Let's try ristretto this time." My friend just bought a Nespresso machine. We were trying different coffee capsules which came with it. I feel coffee coursing through my brain. I already had two shots of espresso (or was it three? Maybe four) from my handcrafted Italian cafetiere before I came over. But who cares! I thought to myself as the machine made gurgling noises and squirted the most wonderful liquid that ever flowed on the face of this godforsaken planet. I could smell it and it tickles my brain. "Ristretto for you my friend!"

Consuming nothing but water for 20 hours or more means quitting coffee or tea. I want to dedicate a chapter on coffee since it's the most popular beverage in the world and since it was the hardest for me to quit. The things we'll discuss about coffee potentially applies to tea since both contain caffeine.

I'm aware of the research on the health benefits of coffee, I was a coffee enthusiast (ahem, addict). Although drinking 8oz. (240 ml.) of black coffee in the morning won't break your prior night's fast, I personally don't recommend drinking coffee anymore.

You absorb caffeine and other organic compounds when you drink coffee.

Coffee is not benign it has metabolic effects. When we don't eat, we want the body to function without external input and rely on its own systems so we get the maximum benefits of food deprivation.

I prefer to play it safe here. In terms of nutrition coffee has little going for it. Aside from trace micronutrients it has little else. It has more disadvantages than advantages from my estimation. From this perspective I thought it would be wiser to quit my coffee habit and in the process save time, money, energy, and mental preoccupation with making good coffee... in addition to not potentially sabotaging what I'm doing with OMAD.

The precise mechanisms at play during food deprivation are not fully understood yet. I prefer to let my body do what it has evolved to do by giving it the conditions which brought about these mechanisms in the first place. Call me an OMAD purist but I think a psychoactive drug like caffeine disrupts these adaptive processes involved in food deprivation.

Caffeine in coffee is the world's most widely used psychoactive drug. It alters brain function and behavior.[90] Caffeine is found in over 60 known plants and it acts as a pesticide in those plants.[91] Consumed by insects, it's lethal. Consumed by humans, we get a buzz.

Caffeine binds to your nerve cells' adenosine receptors. Adenosine comes from your body spending ATP (Adenosine Triphosphate)–a form of energy in the body. The buildup of adenosine in the brain as you spend energy to do work makes you feel tired and drowsy. Caffeine blocks this effect by binding to adenosine receptors, preventing adenosine from binding to those same receptors. More caffeine, less receptors for adenosine to bind to. Instead of slowing down when adenosine sits on the nerve cells, caffeine fires the cells' signals rapidly. The pituitary gland senses those nerves firing rapidly and assumes the brain is in a state of emergency. This molecular maelstrom stimulates the release of adrenaline to prime the body for action, producing the coffee buzz we're all familiar with.[92] This is why one of the common effects of coffee is anxiety, nervousness, agitation, and irritation.

Others may disagree, but I think having the brain in a constant state of emergency can't be good. I just don't want to screw around with the only brain I have.

As with any substance, you'll need more and more to produce the same effects. You can adapt to coffee's wake up aspects but never to its agitation, anxiety, and irritation. In people with anxiety disorders these effects could be more extreme.[93]

Coffee is a stimulant. It raises blood pressure, stimulates the heart, and produces rapid shallow breathing which deprives the brain of the oxygen needed to keep your thinking calm and rational.[94]

As a diuretic, coffee makes you lose water in your body, you urinate more when you drink coffee. Not to mention it makes your armpits sweaty then stinky. Yuck.

Caffeine's half-life is about 5-6 hours. It would take around 5 hours to reduce 200mg of caffeine to 100mg. Another 5 hours to reduce it to 50mg. Then another 5 hours to reduce it to 25mg, so on and so forth... It will take about 7 half-lives or 35 hours before 200mg of caffeine is reduced to 0.781%.[95] Of course, most coffee drinkers don't go more than 35 hours without coffee. It means coffee drinkers are, for lack of better word, constantly caffeinated.

Coffee may also be shifting your biological clock. It delays your 24-hour metabolic rhythm which keeps your body in time with the world.[96] No wonder one of the well-known effect of coffee is disruption of sleep.

Quitting coffee will be hard so I recommend quitting coffee little by little. You can employ the same strategies we used to reduce three meals a day to one meal a day.

I used to drink 2-3 espressos a day, sometimes four. I quit it little by little. First I drank strictly two espresso shots. Then I drank one and a half shot per day, leaving my noon cup half empty. Then I started drinking one at lunchtime. Each time I took my espresso I would consciously leave a little left in the cup. After a while, I've been drinking so little coffee it made sense to just drop the habit. I drank my final cup of coffee before I went on vacation to the Philippines. I used the long transcontinental and transpacific flight to stop the habit. It was hard at first but it got better. Fighting fatigue, sleepiness, lethargy, and inability to concentrate is easier done dozing on planes and airport lounges. When I came back from vacation, I never drank coffee again.

Coffee withdrawal in my experience took 2-3 days before all the symptoms went away, almost the same time as my flight to the Philippines. Fighting withdrawal from coffee also helped me sleep once I landed on the other side of the world, despite the jet lag.

It gets better the longer you don't drink coffee. The first day was the hardest. When the awfulness of coffee withdrawal went away on the third day, I swore to never drink coffee again. It was like being born again when I woke up. Being alert without the need for coffee is a godsend! 2-3 mornings of suffering is nothing compared to a lifetime of dependency and the constant threat of not having a good cup of coffee I got used to in Haiti.

It's hard. I know. But fixing a lifetime of dependency in 2-3 days is a bargain.

Those are the reasons why I don't drink coffee anymore and why I recommend quitting coffee.

Exercise The OMAD Multiplier

I exercise in the afternoon. Exercise depletes glycogen stores quickly so you can start burning fats. It's how I keep my body fat low and looking lean all these years as my cohorts started to get fat and sick. They think getting fat is normal with age, I disagree.

The combination of OMAD and exercise has worked well for me through the years. I may not be big but I'm shredded. I'm also stronger than most people.

If you're doing energy-demanding activities, like marathons and boxing I suggest you eat more and use some supplements. Again, be sensible, if you're losing weight, eat more! OMAD is not gospel.

In terms of exercise you can do whatever exercise you want. Though I advise, if you're just starting with OMAD, avoid intense workouts until you've adapted to OMAD. Start with maybe 25% (or less) of your usual routine. Then increase activity as you get used to a reduced food intake.

If you haven't done any exercises (like most people) get used to OMAD first, then start doing light exercises. Walking is a good place to start. Exercise is important to health, you've heard this a million times before and you know it! So I'm not going to beleaguer the point.

My workout program on OMAD is nothing special and nothing as intense as I used to do. I don't do Crossfit, bodybuilding, or powerlifting anymore. I do simple calisthenic exercises similar to the popular <u>Convict Conditioning by Paul Wade</u>. I do this workout 3x a week then do cardio (running or jump ropes) for half an hour to an hour on the weekends. Sometimes, I run on rest days increasing my exercise frequency to 6 times a week. Here's my simple workout plan in case you want to do it too.

Frequency: 3-5x a week (minimum 3x).

I spend at least 20-30 mins on warm-up: moving my joints, stretching, and doing some yoga positions. Any kind of warm-up routine you like would work. The point is to prepare the body for action little by little.

Do each exercise in proper form. Do 1 set of each exercise with as little rest as possible in between sets. Do all the sets until you finish all the sets.

EXERCISE	# OF SETS	# OF REPETITIONS
Crunches	3x	15-20x
Bridges	3x	10-15x
Calve Raises	3x	10-20x
Squats	3x	10-20x
Pullups	3x	8-10x
Pushups	3x	10-15x

On Saturday and/or Sunday, run or do jump ropes for thirty minutes to an hour.

Some suggests you do stretches for cool down, I don't normally do cool downs. I only do it when I'm training someone else. Usually, walking home after a run or a cold shower after strength training is usually enough for me.

The goal of my exercise program is to keep myself physically fit and strong in addition to maintaining muscle mass. My workout routine can make muscles toned but it's not designed for making muscles Arnold Schwarzenegger big.

This is not an exercise book, so I won't go through how to properly do those exercises or how to do progression exercises. Proper forms for those exercises are easy to search on YouTube.

In the beginning, I suggest to do it with a friend who could check if you're performing the movements properly. You could both watch videos and check each other's form. Better yet, train with a trainer for a month. Have your trainer show you how to do the exercises I mentioned. Remember how it's done so you can do it on yourself once the month with your trainer is up.

It's important to eat something after workout sessions because exercise not only breaks down glycogen and fats, it also breaks down proteins in the muscles.[97] Post-workout consumption of carbohydrates and proteins stimulate improvements in strength and body composition.[98] This is why I prefer to workout and eat at the end of the day.

The body's ability to replenish glycogen stores and rebuild protein is enhanced after exercise. There's a 30-60 minute anabolic window after workouts. Intake of protein and carbohydrates in this time frame will shift the body from a catabolic state (breaking down tissues) to an anabolic state (building tissues).[99] Experts believe the anabolic window is the body's way of overcompensating for the breakdown of proteins and glycogen stores.

It makes plenty of sense to workout at the end of the day, just before eating your one meal. You continuously burn fats during the day and you take advantage of the post-workout eating window.

If your goal is to be strong and have a toned body, exercise is a must. OMAD alone may burn fats, but it won't give you a strong and toned musculature. Think of exercise as a multiplier. The benefits you get from OMAD is multiplied with a proper workout plan.

Take It To Another Level: Fasting

The natural progression of OMAD is fasting. After you've been eating one meal a day for more than a year, I suggest you try a 24-48 hour fast. You can increase to 3-4 days once you're used to two days without food.

I go on a 3-4 day fasts at least once a year. Every quarter if I could manage. To not eat for 4 days and function normally always amazes me, hunger doesn't usually come until the second day then slowly eases on the third day before it disappears. It reminds me of how modern eating habits are really too much, too frequent, and too soon. We're consuming way more than what we need to live. As a result we get sick.

Most benefits of fasting are the same as OMAD. So I won't repeat it here. What's interesting about fasting for more than 24 hours is the process called autophagy—something you don't get with OMAD alone. Exercise also induces autophagy and other protective functions of the cellular pathway.[100] It's another reason for you to exercise. Exercise and OMAD together will get you autophagy. Fasting will give you more benefits in addition to autophagy. Metabolic adaptations happen on a prolonged fast.

Autophagy simply put is your body eating itself. It sounds bad but it isn't. It's a natural highly regulated mechanism which removes the cell's unnecessary or dysfunctional components. This process allows for the orderly degradation and recycling of cellular components.[101] This process is activated by food deprivation (fasting) and exercise. In other words, autophagy is your body's way of cleaning itself and taking out the trash.

One crucial benefit of autophagy is the removal of dysfunctional and unnecessary cellular components which can lead to illness and diseases like cancer. Some studies found autophagy bolsters the immune system. It regulates inflammation[102] and help fight infectious diseases.[103] Autopahgy deficits have also been associated with schizophrenia.[104]

The best benefit of autophagy in my opinion is lifespan extension. It makes you live longer by upregulating natural anti-aging pathways in the body.[105] One of the hallmarks of aging is the accumulation of various molecular damage in the cell, autophagy clears this damage away.

Dr. Jason Fung in his book The Obesity Code says, autophagy is your body taking the oldest, junkiest proteins and burns them for energy. He estimates, the process starts at around 24 hours after your last meal and maximizes at around 32 hours.

In other words, you need to skip eating for 24 hours before the process starts.[106] Then continue without food for at least 32 hours to reap the maximum benefits of autophagy. Adding physical activity or exercise can induce autophagy sooner because exercise depletes the body's glycogen stores.

When you start fasting the same principles apply. Do it slowly. First go on a 24-hour fast, then add more time as you get used to it. I don't recommend going longer than 4-5 days. Food deprivation though beneficial is stressful to the body. Anything longer than 5 days may require medical supervision, especially if your health is less than perfect.

After 4-5 days of not eating, start slow. I usually start with a piece of fruit or some cooked vegetables. Then I eat as usual. Nothing special. I treat a fast the same way as I would treat OMAD. You can also have a glass of water tinged with citrus fruit or apple cider vinegar to increase stomach acidity.

During the fasting period I try not to do anything stressful. I skip my workouts. I usually use the fasting period to relax and reflect on life. I binge watch on the series I never normally have time to watch. I read a good book. I meditate.

Remember to drink plenty of water when you're fasting. Water is the only thing you'll consume in the next few days, so drink up more than normal! If you're hungry drink warm water, I find it helps. Especially because you'll feel cold when you fast—it's your body conserving energy for other vital functions.

Salt is important, we lose salt as we go through the day. Since you're consuming nothing for the next 3-4 days, add a pinch of salt on your drinking water.

MUSHROOM OMELETTE

Serves: 1

Prep Time: 5 Minutes

Cook Time: 10 Minutes

Total Time:15Minutes

INGREDIENTS

2 eggs

¼ tsp salt

¼ tsp black pepper

1 tablespoon olive oil

¼ cup cheese

¼ tsp basil

1 cup mushrooms

DIRECTIONS

1.In a bowl combine all ingredients together and mix well

2.In a skillet heat olive oil and pour the egg mixture

3.Cook for 1-2 minutes per side

4.When ready remove omelette from the skillet and serve

PUMPKIN OMELETTE

Serves: 1

Prep Time: 5 Minutes

Cook Time: 10 Minutes

Total Time:15Minutes

INGREDIENTS

2 eggs

¼ tsp salt

¼ tsp black pepper

1 tablespoon olive oil

¼ cup cheese

¼ tsp basil

1 cup pumpkin puree

DIRECTIONS

1.In a bowl combine all ingredients together and mix well

2.In a skillet heat olive oil and pour the egg mixture

3.Cook for 1-2 minutes per side

4.When ready remove omelette from the skillet and serve

BLUEBERRIES OATMEAL

Serves: 2

Prep Time: 10 Minutes

Cook Time: 8 Hours

Total Time:8Hours

INGREDIENTS

1/3 cup oats

1/3 cup blueberries

2 tbs maple syrup

1/3 cup coconut milk

½ tsp vanilla

1 banana

1 ½ tsp chia seeds

DIRECTIONS

1.Mix the oats and chia seeds together

2.Pour in the milk and top with blueberries and sliced banana

3.Refrigerate for at least 8 hours

4.Stir in the maple syrup and serve

CHIA PUDDING

Serves: 2

Prep Time: 5 Minutes

Cook Time: 10 Minutes

Total Time:15Minutes

INGREDIENTS

5 tbs chia seeds

1 ½ tbs vanilla

2 tbs maple syrup

2 ½ cup almond milk

1 ½ cup strawberries

1 beet

DIRECTIONS

1.Blend together the milk, strawberries, chopped beet, maple syrup, and vanilla

2.Pour into a cup and ad the chia

3.Stir every 5 minutes for 15 minutes

4.Refrigerate overnight

5.Serve topped with fruits

BREAKFAST CASSEROLE

Serves: 4

Prep Time: 10 Minutes

Cook Time: 35 Minutes

Total Time:45Minutes

INGREDIENTS

7 oz asparagus

3 tbs parsley

1 cup broccoli

1 zucchini

3 tbs oil

5 eggs

Salt

Pepper

DIRECTIONS

1.Cook the diced zucchini, asparagus and broccoli florets in heated oil for about 5 minutes

2.Season with salt and pepper and remove from heat

3.Whisk the eggs and season then add the parsley

4.Place the vegetables in a greased pan then pour the eggs over

5.Bake in the preheated oven for about 35 minutes at 350F

BLUEBERRY BALLS

Serves: 12

Prep Time: 5 Minutes

Cook Time: 30 Minutes

Total Time:35Minutes

INGREDIENTS

2 cups oats

1 cup blueberries

1/3 cup honey

1 tsp cinnamon

1 ½ tsp vanilla

1/3 cup almond butter

DIRECTIONS

1.Mix the honey, vanilla, oats, almond butter, and cinnamon together

2.Fold in the blueberries

3.Refrigerate for at least 30 minutes

4.Form balls from the dough and serve

ZUCCHINI BREAD

Serves: 4

Prep Time: 10 Minutes

Cook Time: 40 Minutes

Total Time:50Minutes

INGREDIENTS

4 tbs honey

5 tbs oil

1 ½ tsp baking soda

3 eggs

½ cup walnuts

2 ½ cups flour

4 Medjool dates

1 banana

2 tsp mixed spice

1 ½ cup zucchini

DIRECTIONS

1.Preheat the oven to 350 F

2.Chop the dates and the walnuts

3.Mix the flour, spice and baking soda together

4.Mix the eggs and banana in a food processor then add remaining ingredients and mix

5.Pour the batter into a pan and cook for at least 40 minutes

6.Allow to cool then serve